*

Obstetric Forceps

Obstetric Forceps

Leonard E. Laufe, M.D., F.A.C.O.G.

Chief, Division of Obstetrics and Gynecology
The Western Pennsylvania Hospital
Pittsburgh

Assisted by Raymond J. Cristina, M. Litt.

WITH 97 ILLUSTRATIONS

HOEBER MEDICAL DIVISION
Harper & Row, Publishers
New York, Evanston, and London

Library of Congress catalog card number: 68-29056
Designed by The Etheredges

*

To my three patient women—
Sy, Lucy and Jenny

Contents

*

Preface

*

This book is intended for both the resident in obstetrics and gynecology and the practicing obstetrician. It is my hope that it will serve as a handbook on the use of obstetric forceps.

The volume of knowledge related to our specialty increases at an explosive rate—in our affluent society it is fashionable to pursue what is new. A significant sign of the times is our tendency to forget that the purpose of graduate training is to produce competent clinicians whose prime concern must be the care of patients. As physicians, they must not merely function, but function well, in both the delivery and operating rooms. Graduate training programs, therefore, should emphasize the clinical fundamentals of the specialty.

Since the forces of labor, application of forceps, and delivery of the infant are such dynamic subjects, every teaching aid must be employed if the student is to fully comprehend them. The classroom lecture and the use of the mannikin can provide the student with theoretic knowledge but the ultimate learning experience is the demonstration and use of the forceps in the delivery room. The final goal of forceps instruction cannot be taught by implication but must be achieved by the student himself.

One of the essentials in teaching the use of obstetric forceps is to instill a respect for the various instruments and the values, indications, and limitations of each. They are not "hooks" or "claws" but surgical instruments. They are not for "spinning" or "dragging" but assist in rotation and extraction. Proportionately larger than most surgical instruments, they are involved with a most sensitive object. Their use must be approached with the same temerity as is any surgical procedure and with an adherence to sound surgical principles.

Proper instruction regarding obstetric forceps must be predicated on a sound knowledge of the forces of labor, the anatomy of the female pelvis, and the positions the fetus can assume. When these are appreciated, the factors which contribute or predispose to a particular problem are understood. Only then can a proper instrument be selected for use. Just as we try to cultivate surgical judgment in our training programs, we should encourage "forceps" judgment.

Familiarity, in this instance, fosters respect. If the student is to properly use an instrument, he must be comfortable with it. Aware of the origin, construction, and functions of a forceps, he then can appreciate the forces involved. As new or modified instruments appear, he will be in a position to consider and evaluate them.

I have attempted to confine this book to that material which is pertinent to the proper *use* of obstetric forces. For this reason, I have intentionally avoided any discussion of version and extraction or the vacuum extractor. Version seems to have finally found its limited place as an operative procedure, while the vacuum extractor is being thoroughly discussed in the current literature. I have tried to limit the content to those forceps and procedures which are most commonly employed today. Included are brief clinical backgrounds of the various problems for which forceps are indicated. Finally, I have assumed that the reader has a basic knowledge of obstetrics and have tried to avoid repetitious description of technic.

This book could not have been written without the wonderful wealth of literature upon which I was able to draw. Especially useful have been the works of Das, Dennen, and the symposia *Clinical Obstetrics and Gynecology*.

I am particularly indebted to the J. Sklar Manufacturing Co., Inc., Long Island City, N.Y., who have been kind enough to help me with my modifications of obstetric forceps and who provided the drawings of forceps which have been liberally used throughout the text. The C. V. Mosby Company, St. Louis, Missouri, generously allowed me to extract considerable historical material from Das.

Many are responsible for this endeavor. My former Chief, Dr. H. A. Power, encouraged my early interest in obstetric forceps. My residents provided the impetus to record our forceps seminars. My associate, Dr. John L. Ammer, contributed considerable patience while this book was being prepared.

Mr. John Vetter supervised the art work and photography. Miss Michele Ryan did the line drawings. Miss Donna Harris has faithfully typed and retyped manuscript. Mr. Frank Stark helped me to understand the mechanical principles of obstetric forceps. Many others have assisted in a variety of ways. I am also most grateful to my publisher, the Hoeber Medical Division of Harper & Row, and particularly to Mrs. Eunice Stevens, my editor, and also to Miss Jo Hinkel.

LEONARD E. LAUFE, M.D.

Pittsburgh, Pennsylvania

*

Obstetric Forceps

*

Chapter One

The Evolution of Obstetric Forceps

THE ANCIENTS

The obstetric forceps is a unique instrument. A simple and honest implement, compared to many of man's inventions, its history is nevertheless complicated with confusion and irony and its invention shrouded in secrecy. It probably has saved more lives than any instrument ever devised, and yet it did not appear until countless generations of men struggled into the world without it, or failed to arrive. A real and solid thing, easily fabricated, it is yet capable of such subtle variation that its evolution has never stopped. It is designed specifically to rescue life, and yet it descended from an instrument of death.

The ancients had various instruments to which they resorted when normal delivery was impossible, but by their very nature, these instruments were not capable of bringing forth a child alive. They were tools of mutilation, and they were used in an attempt to save the life of the mother only.

Hindu writings of a thousand years before Christ refer to a knife and a hook resorted to in difficult labors. The knife was used to perforate the head, and the hook to extract the dead fetus.

Hippocrates dealt with the matter of difficult labor in his writings of 400 B.C., but the only instruments referred to were those for the mutilation and extraction of a child already dead.

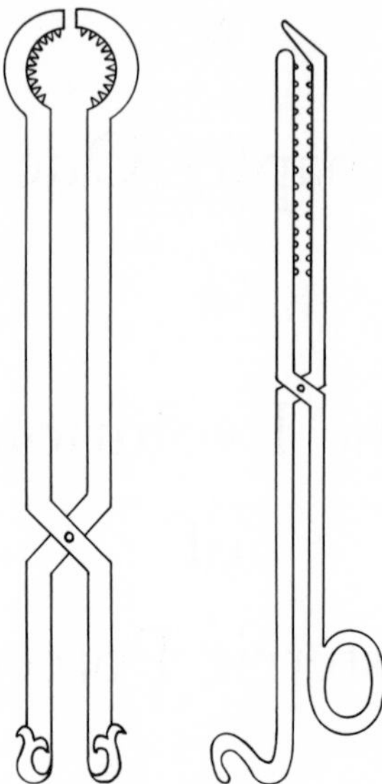

Fig. 1-1. Forceps of Albucasis. *(Adapted from Das: Obstetric Forceps, St. Louis, 1929, The C. V. Mosby Company.)*

Soranus, the eminent Greek physician of the early second century A.D., wrote a significant *Gynecology*. In it, he explains the role of the midwife: "Now she must insert the fingers gently at the time of dilation and pull the fetus forward, giving way when the uterus draws itself together, but pulling lightly when it dilates." When human hands failed to deliver the infant safely, however, the only alternative was the usual, drastic one: "If the fetus does not respond to manual traction, because of its size, or death, or impaction in any manner whatsoever, one must proceed to the more forceful methods, those of extraction by hooks and embryotomy. For even if one loses the infant, it is still necessary to take care of the mother." There, succinctly stated, is the concept of midwifery from the time of the ancients until the seventeenth century and the Chamberlen era.

Perhaps only one man of these early times, the celebrated Arabian obstetrician, Avicenna, approached the concept of a saving forceps. Drawings of the obstetric forceps of that time by his contemporary, Albucasis, about 1000 A.D., show a number of crushing implements with murderous teeth (Fig. 1-1). None of these could have delivered a living child, unless it be terribly mutilated. But there is a passage in the writing of Avicenna which leaves open the possibility, however remote, that another kind of obstetric forceps may have existed.

Avicenna[22] wrote that if manual traction is not successful, it should be followed by use of the fillet, a net or cloth band worked over the head of the fetus by which the infant might be forcibly withdrawn. If the fillet is unsuccessful, he continues, then "let the forceps be applied, and let it be delivered by them." Significantly, Avicenna adds that should the forceps be unsuccessful, the infant must be withdrawn by incision "as in the case of a dead fetus." Does the sequence of these statements imply that the forceps, coming as it does before the last alternative, might be used to deliver a child *alive?*

It is a slim possibility which has supported much speculation through the ages. If Avicenna did, indeed, possess a conservative forceps, the instrument was thereafter lost to knowledge, and only his provocative phrasing remains to suggest that it might once have existed.

Historical speculation supports one other figure before the Chamberlens as the possible inventor of a conservative forceps. Jacob Rueff,[22] the city physician of Zurich, presented in his *Midwifery* of 1554 a drawing of a smooth-bladed instrument which was conserva-

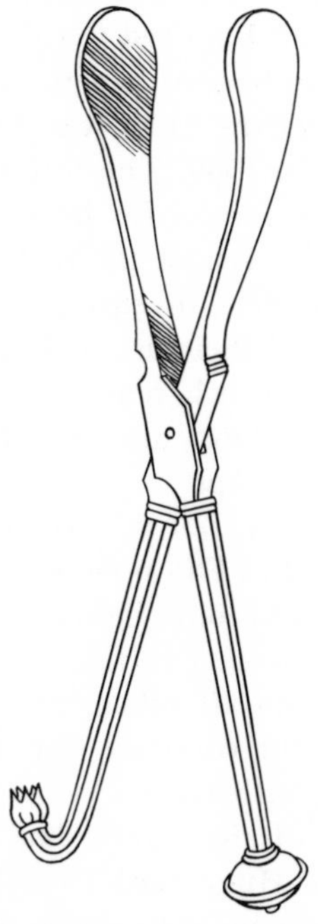

Fig. 1-2. Forceps of Rueff. *(Adapted from Das: Obstetric Forceps, St. Louis, 1929, The C. V. Mosby Company.)*

tive at least in appearance. It is a locked pincers, crossed at the shanks, with cup-shaped ends instead of teeth (Fig. 1-2). It bears more resemblance to a lithotomy forceps, however, than to the obstetric forceps developed in England early in the next century. Because of its rigid construction, it is doubtful that this instrument could have been manipulated to accomplish a live delivery. More likely it was used in the extraction of a dead fetus, for the drawing illustrates a chapter entitled, "How and with what instruments children sticking in the wombe, and being dead, are to be brought forth."

THE CHAMBERLENS

The turn of the century brought into existence, finally, the first truly conservative obstetric forceps—an instrument capable of saving the life of the infant as well as that of the mother. Credit for its invention must go to one of a remarkable family of physicians, the Chamberlens, practicing in England during the whole of the seventeenth century. Which of the Chamberlens actually invented the instrument will never be known for certain. Paradoxically, after mankind's long wait for this urgently needed device, it was kept a family secret for more than a hundred years!

Four generations of Chamberlens practiced midwifery in England between 1600 and 1728. Peter the Elder was the first, having emigrated with his father from Paris in 1569. The forceps might very well have originated with him, accounting for his fame as an accoucheur. Hugh Chamberlen, Junior, was the last of the male heirs, and by the time he died in 1728, the independent invention of forceps by obstetricians outside the family had spread their use in England and abroad.

But for most of the seventeenth century, if not for all of it, three Peter Chamberlens, a Paul, a John, and two Hugh Chamberlens had a monopoly on the obstetric forceps.

As Hugh Chamberlen, Senior, put it,[22] writing in the 1670's, ". . . My Father, Brothers, and my Self, (Tho none else in Europe that I know) have, by God's Blessing, and our Industry, attained to, and long practised a way to deliver Women in this case, without any prejudice to them or their Infants; tho all others (being obliged, for want of such an Expedient, to use the common way) do, and must endanger, if not destroy one or both, with Hooks."

By this time, the fame of the family had spread throughout the country and the Continent. Hugh Senior's father, Dr. Peter Chamberlen, had acted as "Physician in ordinary to three Kings and Queens of England," according to the epitaph on his tomb in Woodham.

It was in Woodham, at the former estate of Dr. Peter Chamberlen of the Court of England, that several models of the Chamberlen forceps were actually found. They were discovered purely by accident in a secret receptacle under the floor of a closet, among a collection of old coins and trinkets. The date of the discovery was June, 1813—some 200 years after their invention.

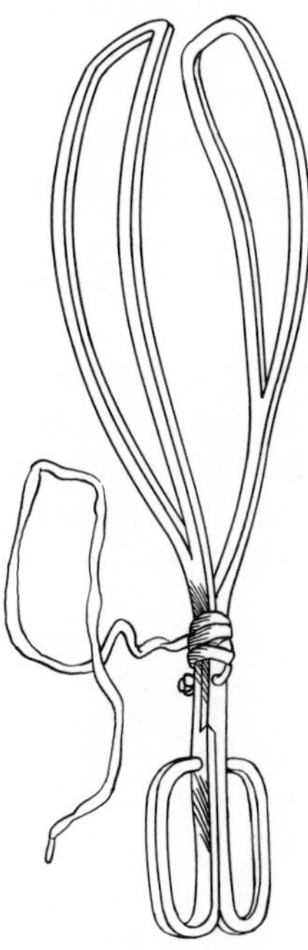

Fig. 1-3. Chamberlen forceps. *(Adapted from Das: Obstetric Forceps, St. Louis, 1929, The C. V. Mosby Company.)*

What was the construction of these carefully hidden instruments—simple, but effective. The blades were fenestrated and had a cephalic curve. The branches—about 12 in. long—crossed in the manner of a pair of scissors. They could be separated at the shanks for insertion one at a time, then be rejoined with either a rivet or a thong (Fig. 1-3).

The fact that the blades were separable was the key to the success of the forceps. This same feature, incidentally, permitted Hugh Chamberlen, Senior, to sell one-half the pair to Rogier Roonhuyse, it is said, when the English physician retired to Holland late in life. Roonhuyse's "lever" passed to other hands and for a while was widely used in Holland.

It cannot be shown that any other disclosure of the Chamberlen forceps was ever made, and the family has been censured by many historians for guarding the instrument so zealously and for so long. More tolerant writers point out, however, that trade secrets were not uncommon among medical practitioners of the day and that the Chamberlens were no worse than their neighbors, but only more inventive.

The inventive genius of other obstetricians was not long denied after the demise of the last Chamberlen. By the middle of the eighteenth century, this inventiveness and a better understanding of the mechanism of labor had produced the forceps of Palfyn, Dusée, Giffard, Chapman, Pugh, Levret, and Smellie.

THE EARLY INNOVATORS

The first important innovation was made by Dusée of France. He flattened the shanks of his forceps where they crossed and joined them with a removable screw. Better locking devices evolved, of course, but this method of articulation influenced the design of French and German forceps thereafter (Fig. 1-4).

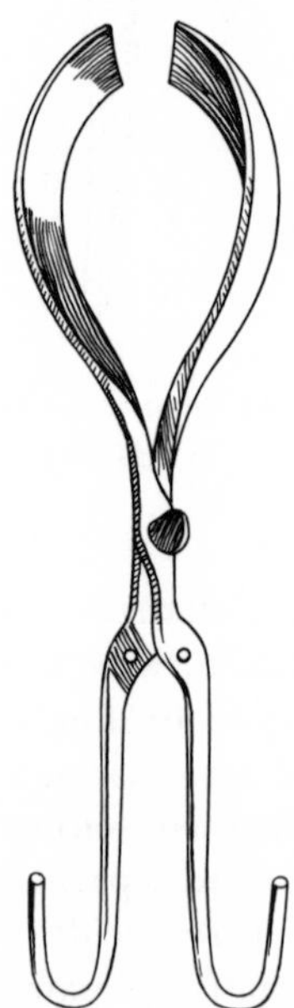

Fig. 1-4. Forceps of Dusée. *(Adapted from Das: Obstetric Forceps, St. Louis, 1929, The C. V. Mosby Company.)*

The most valuable improvement was the development of the pelvic curve by Pugh, Levret, and Smellie within a few years of one another. Levret was the first to give a public account of this modification, which he did before the Royal Academy of Surgery of Paris in 1747. His purpose in adding the pelvic curve, he explained, was to avoid injury to the perineum. It was the first instrumental variation aimed distinctly at reducing trauma to the mother. Smellie's goal was an instrument which could reach the head of the fetus while it was still high in the pelvis.

The two men may have had different objectives in mind, but the addition of the pelvic curve to the cephalic curve resulted in a forceps which was considerably advanced beyond that of the Chamberlens. With the presence of handles, shanks, and the two major curves plus a locking mechanism to join the branches, the essential design of the modern obstetric forceps had been achieved.

The next one hundred years produced a plethora of obstetric forceps. Some instruments represented no more than slight variations on already accepted principles of forceps construction. Others represented ingenious but futile attempts to obtain higher and easier forceps applications, better grasp of the fetal head, and improved traction. There were instruments with detachable blades or detachable handles; forceps whose blades moved in the horizontal plane and forceps whose blades moved in the vertical; forceps with movable shanks and flexible handles; forceps with levers and forceps with pulleys. There were even attempts to make forceps of leather or wood, but the impossibility of keeping the instruments clean and controlling the cumulative stench precluded their continued use.

Despite all this experimentation, little progress was made against the problems of fetal and maternal damage. It remained popular during this century of forceps development to utilize the ends of the handles for perforators and hooks should the instrument fail in extraction. Yet assertions regarding the effect of the injudicious use of forceps had been repeatedly voiced. None stated it more aptly than Benjamin Bell. In his *A System of Surgery* in 1789 he wrote, "By not meeting with the attention which it merits, both the forceps and crotchet are daily employed with too much freedom to the disgrace of the art, and often with irreparable injury to the mother and child." And as late as the 1800's Professor Pajot, a most respected authority of the day, still found it necessary to warn his students that the perforator and hook at the ends of the handles were there as a reminder that they should never be used.

THE MODERN INNOVATORS

It wasn't until the latter half of the nineteenth century—with Kristeller, Tarnier, Simpson, and Elliott—that a better understanding of the function of obstetric forceps was achieved. With this understanding came efforts to reduce the potential dangers of the forceps.

Kristeller was the first to attempt the scientific measurement of the extractile force employed in the use of forceps. He devised a dynamometrical apparatus adapted to the handle of the instrument. In essence, the handle contained a spiral spring which was compressed with traction. The compression of the spring was reflected in a sliding metric scale on the surface of the handle. The reading of compression obtained when the forceps was used was then converted to the force applied.

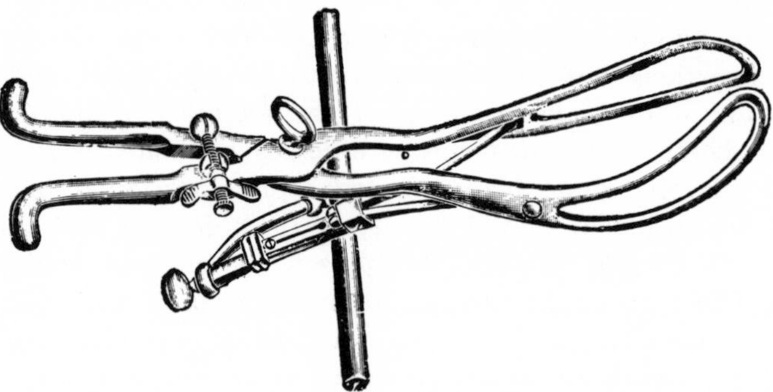

Fig. 1-5. Forceps of Tarnier. *(Courtesy of J. Sklar Manufacturing Company.)*

The greatest contribution to the improvement of the obstetric forceps during the nineteenth century came from Tarnier.[101-103] This Frenchman, Pajot's successor, had already achieved fame for his monograph on puerperal fever. From 1877 to 1881 he developed and refined an axis-traction forceps. His work was based on the forceps of Morales, who in 1864 presented to the Belgium Academy of Medicine an instrument with a perineal curve in the shanks and handles in order to obtain perfect traction.

The criteria which Tarnier's instrument was to fulfill were: (*1*) constant and easy traction along the axis of the pelvic planes; (*2*) freedom of rotary movement of the fetal head through the pelvis; and (*3*) the presence of an indicator which would constantly inform the operator of the desired direction of traction (Fig. 1-5).

Tarnier's forceps is the prototype of innumerable traction instruments which have subsequently appeared, and his theory of axis-traction is responsible for the development of the popular axis-traction handle developed by Bill for use with conventional forceps.

Shortly before Tarnier's monumental contribution, James Simpson of Edinburgh was perfecting his forceps, which still retain much popularity. He was an impressive personality and world-renowned for his use of chloroform. In 1848 he described his long and short forceps, with emphasis on traction rather than compression. He utilized a long tapered blade for better adaptation to the molded fetal head and a loose simple lock. The parallel shanks parted above the lock sufficiently to allow a finger to be placed between them, which was an aid in reducing compression (Fig. 1-6).

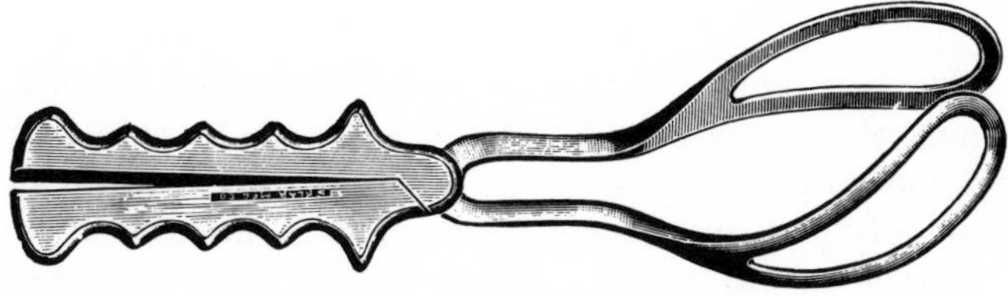

Fig. 1-6. Forceps of Simpson. *(Courtesy of J. Sklar Manufacturing Company.)*

A decade later Elliott of New York introduced his forceps and reiterated the necessity of avoiding compression. He devised an adjustable pin within the handles as a means of regulating lateral pressure. Elliott's forceps had shorter blades with an increased cephalic curve, as compared to Simpson's, and also possessed overlapping rather than parallel shanks (Fig. 1-7).

These two forceps, the Simpson and the Elliott, became the prototypes of the most frequently used outlet forceps. Subtle modifications of these instruments have been subsequently made by DeLee and others but their basic architecture has remained intact.

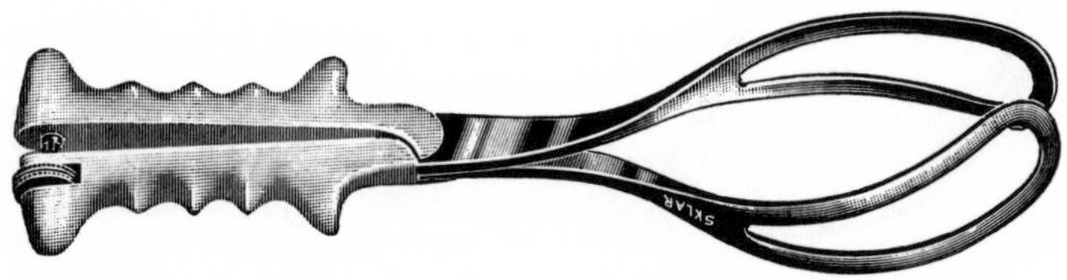

Fig. 1-7. Forceps of Elliott. *(Courtesy of J. Sklar Manufacturing Company.)*

The concept of solid nonfenestrated blades for easier application and removal led to their reappearance in the latter half of the nineteenth century. Knight, Olshausen, and McLane each introduced forceps with such blades. It wasn't until 1937, however, that Luikart[58] refined this modification to its present popular state.

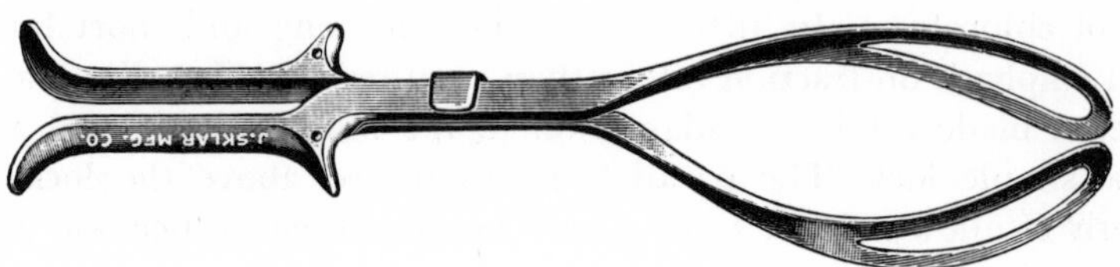

Fig. 1-8. Forceps of Kielland. *(Courtesy of J. Sklar Manufacturing Company.)*

The most ingenious and perhaps best constructed forceps among those commonly employed today is the Kielland. Introduced in 1915 and originally intended for deep transverse arrests, it probably is the most commonly used instrument for midpelvic rotations. The instrument is unique in possessing a sliding lock to allow for asynclytism, directional markers on the handles for orientation toward the occiput, and negation of the pelvic curve by an altered angulation of the shanks and handles with the blades. This gives the instrument a bayonet shape (Fig. 1-8).

The most unique appearing of the forceps in current use is that designed by Lyman Barton of Plattsburg, New York (Fig. 1-9). He was an imaginative practitioner who conceived his instrument some twenty years before it was formally introduced before the New York Obstetrical Society in 1925. Although Uytterhoven in 1805, Baumers in 1849, and Cameron in 1893 had designed forceps which were to be applied

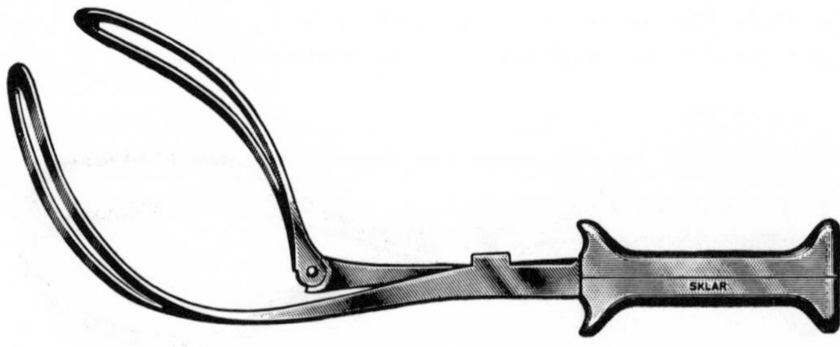

Fig. 1-9. Forceps of Barton. *(Courtesy of J. Sklar Manufacturing Company.)*

in the anteroposterior pelvic planes, Barton apparently was unaware of their efforts. These instruments never achieved popularity because of their rigidity, which made the retropubic blade difficult to apply.

Barton's forceps is successful for traction of a transverse arrest in the transverse pelvic plane because of the anterior hinged blade and the 50° angulation of the shanks and blades. The instrument also has a sliding lock, although Barton was unaware of Kielland's instrument. A special traction bar can also be employed with this forceps.

The need for a suitable instrument for the management of the aftercoming head was first recognized by Piper. His long forceps with tapered blades, parallel shanks, and a marked perineal curve has become a standard instrument in all delivery rooms (Fig. 1-10).

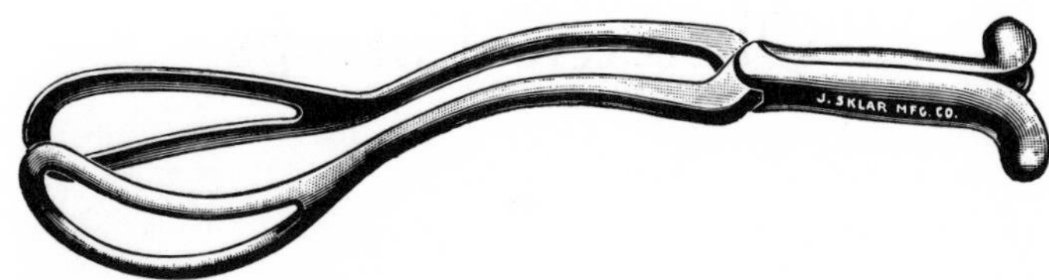

Fig. 1-10. Forceps of Piper. *(Courtesy of J. Sklar Manufacturing Company.)*

The Simpson and Elliott forceps and their subsequent modifications, such as the Tucker-McLane, represent the most commonly used obstetric forceps of today. The Bill traction handle, which adds instrumental axis-traction to any of the conventional forceps, has become a popular adjunct. Of the forceps designed with an integral axis-traction handle, the Dewey is probably the most frequently employed. The Kielland, Barton, and Piper are the special instruments which complete the usual armamentarium of the practicing obstetrician.

Although the evolution of the obstetric forceps continues, and each year new instruments appear, none of the newer forceps has yet achieved sufficient popularity or been subjected to adequate trial to warrant inclusion in this brief history.

*

Chapter Two

*

The Anatomy of Obstetric Forceps

Forceps can be separated into different groups by numerous methods of classification. They can be divided according to length (short and long forceps), shape (straight and curved forceps), function (rotation and outlet forceps), or even by geographic or historic determinations. The most meaningful system, however, is classification according to the method of articulation.

Das has neatly categorized obstetric forceps into four groups based on the relationship of the branches. The branches either cross in the shape of an X, diverge in the shape of a V, are parallel, or converge toward the toes of the blades (Fig. 2-1). The last group of instruments is of historical interest only. Parallel forceps of antiquity are those of Palfyn, while modern examples are the spatulas of Thierry and the parallel forceps of Shute.

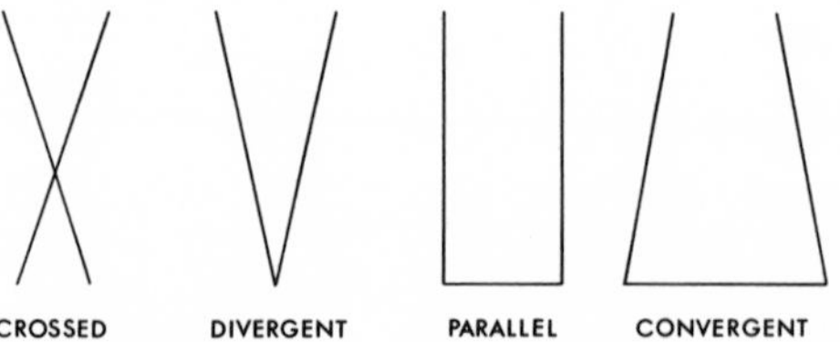

Fig. 2-1. Types of forceps. *(Adapted from Das: Obstetric Forceps, St. Louis, 1929, The C. V. Mosby Company.)*

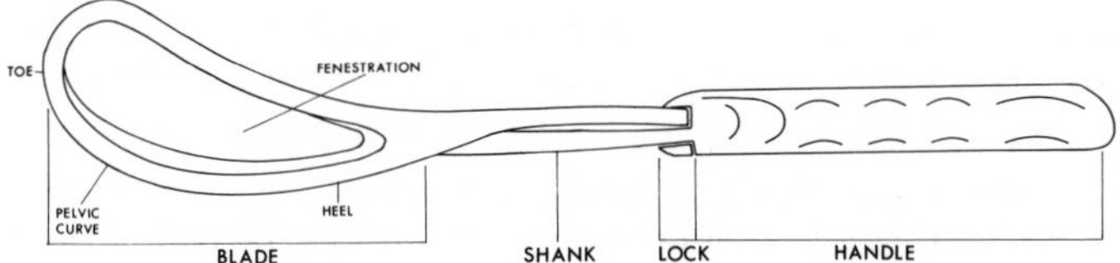

Fig. 2-2. Anatomy of obstetric forceps (lateral view).

Most obstetric forceps in common use descend from the Chamberlen instrument and exemplify the cross or scissors construction with the fulcrum near the middle of the X. The first forceps with divergent branches was introduced in 1781 by Thenance. Unfortunately, Thenance's forceps was excessively long and unwieldy, and the principle of divergence was discarded along with the instrument. Boerma in 1907 inadvertently utilized the principle of divergence in the design of his forceps, but he included indentations on the parallel shanks of his instrument to encourage compression. His forceps, too, was looked upon with disfavor.

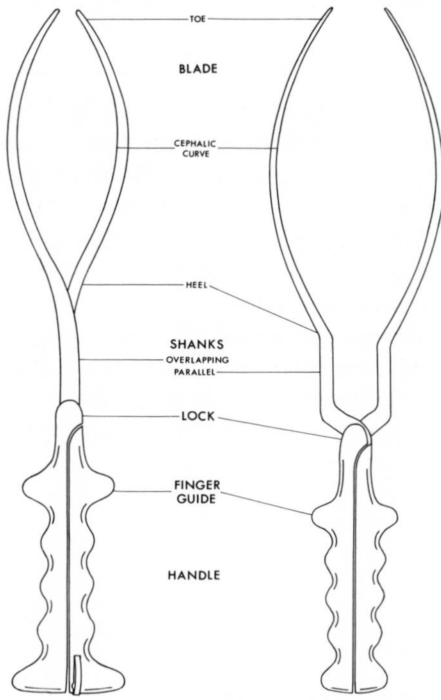

Figure 2-3. Anatomy of Elliott (*left*) and Simpson (*right*) obstetric forceps (superior view).

Although the concept of divergence has never achieved any popularity, it deserves renewed consideration as a means of controlling the compressive force. Forceps designed in the divergent principle function as third-class levers and, when properly used, exert no direct compressive force to the fetal head. The author is attempting to revive interest in divergent forceps with his modifications of the Piper instrument[56] and outlet forceps.[57]

All obstetric forceps have the same fundamental components. Each has two branches, or vecti, designated right or left by their orientation to the pelvic walls. With conventional crossed forceps, the left branch is applied to the left side of the pelvis and the handle fits the operator's left hand. With parallel or divergent instruments, the branches do not cross and hence the left branch fits the operator's right hand. Each branch consists of three major parts: the blade, which relates to the fetal head and maternal pelvis; the handle, with which the operator manipulates the instrument; and the shank, which is the portion of each branch between the blade and handle. Each branch articulates with its mate by a locking mechanism which is usually located at or near the junction of the shanks and handles (Figs. 2-2 and 2-3).

BLADES

The blades of obstetric forceps possess two basic curves. The *cephalic* curve is concave and designed to fit the lateral convexity of the fetal head. The *pelvic* curve corresponds to the descending curve of the maternal pelvis. These primary curves of the obstetric blades are subtly varied by the blade length and by the construction of the individual instrument. The pelvic curve can also be influenced by the angle with which the shank joins the blade.

The two curves maintain a fixed 90° relationship to each other, with one exception. The exclusive instrument is the Barton forceps. When applied in the anteroposterior plane of the pelvis to a transverse arrest, the cephalic and pelvic curves of the posterior blade are parallel (Fig. 2-4).

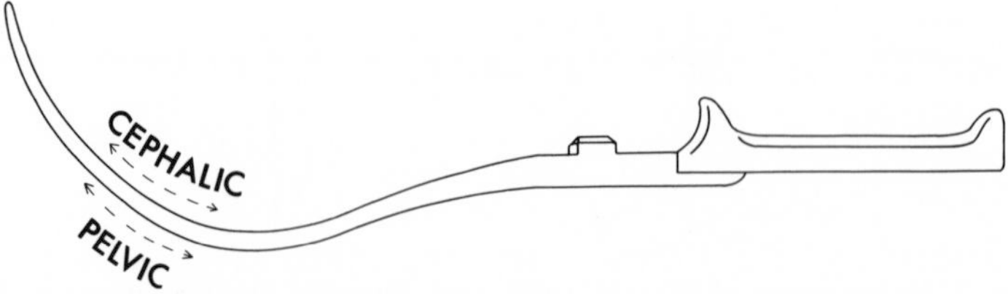

Fig. 2-4. Parallel pelvic and cephalic curves of Barton forceps.

The blades of obstetric forceps have two basic lengths. The Simpson forceps and its related types have blades which are 18 cm. long. The short Elliott-type forceps, which include the Tucker-McLane and Luikart instruments, have 15-cm. blades. In the Simpson group, the blades are more tapered; when their branches are articulated and approximated, the toes of the bades are 3.5 cm. apart. In the short Elliott-type instrument, Tucker-McLane, and Kielland, the toes are 1.5 cm. apart. The long Elliott forceps has 18-cm. blades which are separated 2.5 cm. at their toes (*see* Fig. 2-3).

Blade breadth and contour also vary among the instruments. Most blades have an eccentric contour, being narrow at the heel and gradually widening to a breadth of 5 cm. as the toe is approached and the pelvic curve reaches its peak (*see* Fig. 2-2). The blades of the Kielland forceps are only 4 cm. in breadth. The instruments which have symmetrical blades are the Barton and its modifications, since they were designed for application to the anteroposterior diameter of the pelvis rather than to the transverse.

Most of the obstetric forceps in common use have blades of approximately 3-mm. thickness. The prime exception is the Kielland. The inner surface of its blade is slightly convex, giving it a beveled contour and thus making the blade slightly thicker. The purpose of this increased thickness is to afford a better grasp of the fetal head for rotation. This feature has been included in the Hawks-Dennen forceps.

Prior to 1937, and with the exception of a few of the early prototypes, most obstetric forceps had fenestrated blades. Size of the fenestration varies, depending upon the shape of the blade, but the rim surrounding the fenestration usually is 8 mm. in breadth.

The Tucker-McLane forceps was the first instrument with solid blades to achieve popularity in modern times. Advocates of the instrument emphasized the ease of application and removal of the blade. There are no internal edges to either hook onto the fetal ear or traumatize the tissues. The solid-blade concept reached its peak of refinement, however, with Luikart's modification.[58] He produced a "pseudofenestration" by decreasing the thickness of the blade at the former site of fenestration. This combined the easy applicability of a solid blade with the firm grip of a fenestrated one. Most obstetric forceps which are being produced today are available with Luikart's modification.

SHANKS

The shanks of the various obstetric forceps in common use also show considerable variation. Their length varies from 4 cm. in short outlet forceps such as the Simpson or short Elliott to a maximum length of 15 cm. in the Piper. Usually, the longer the shank, the longer the instrument. This implies increased leverage and increased force. It was the purpose of those men who modified instruments by shortening their shanks to limit the amount of traction which could be applied.

Shanks of the Simpson group of instruments are parallel and 2.2 cm. apart. They diverge abruptly beyond the lock. The space between them allows the middle finger to be inserted, somewhat as a cushion, in order to aid in minimizing compression (*see* Fig. 2-3).

The Elliott-type forceps, the Kielland, Barton and the Kielland-Barton (K-B) forceps all have overlapping shanks. As with the Simpson, the shank is basically rectangular in shape but gradually tapers as it approaches the blade.

The shanks of the classic and modified Piper forceps are parallel, as with the Simpson type instruments, but are cylindrical in contour. Because of their great length, the cylindrical parallel shanks of the long Piper forceps impart a springlike quality to the instrument.

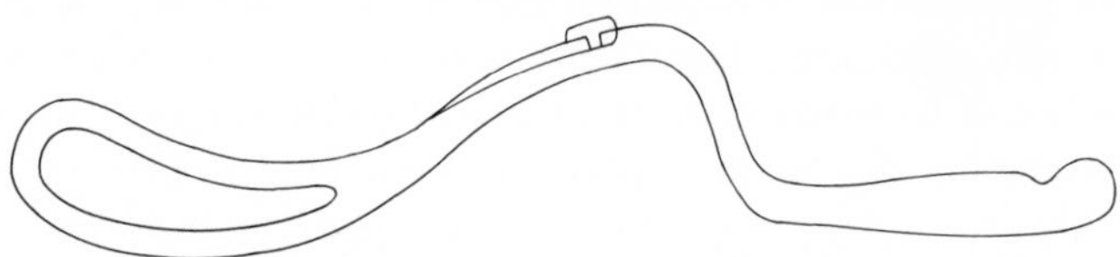

Fig. 2-5. Forceps of Morales. *(Adapted from Das: Obstetric Forceps, St. Louis, 1929, The C. V. Mosby Company.)*

During the past one hundred years, a third curve within the shank of the obstetric forceps has evolved. Hubert was the first to realize the value of this addition. The perineal curve which he imparted to the shanks of his instruments was further accentuated by Morales (Fig. 2-5). On the basis of the latter's forceps, Tarnier brought the concept of axis-traction through a perineal curve to fruition. Although not curved, the Hawks-Dennen forceps employs the same principle by way of the angle with which the blade and shank join.

The relationship of the shank with the blade is of utmost importance. When most conventional instruments are placed upon a flat surface, the pelvic curve becomes obvious as the toes of the blades rise from the horizontal. This is not true of the Kielland forceps. When the handles and shanks of this instrument are on a flat surface, the blades dip beneath the horizontal. If one takes a branch of the Kielland, however, and holds the blade in parallel approximation to the blade of an Elliott forceps, their similar contour is obvious. Ac-

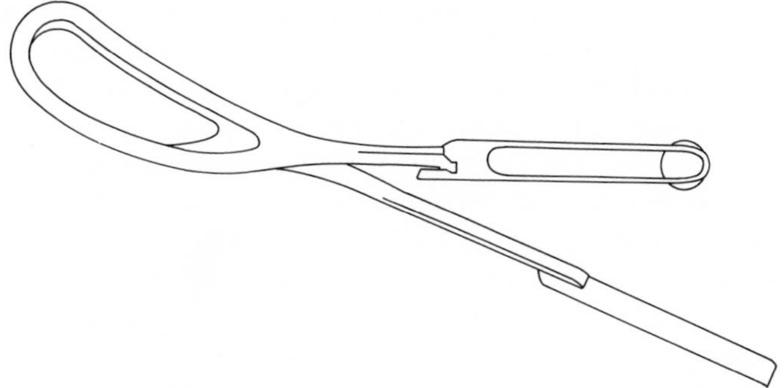

Fig. 2-6. Relationship of shank and blade of conventional and Kielland forceps.

tually it is the angle at which the shank and blade join which reverses the functional curve of the Kielland (Fig. 2-6).

Another instrument with a unique angle of the shanks and blades is the Barton forceps. The blades extend from the shanks at a 50° angle. A second distinguishing feature of the Barton, which has also been employed in the Kielland-Barton forceps (K-B), is the presence of a hinged blade.

LOCKS

The locks of obstetric forceps have an intriguing history in themselves. The early locks were named after the schools of teaching from which they originated. These are the English, French, and German. The more recently devised locking mechanisms have descriptive titles such as sliding or pivot.

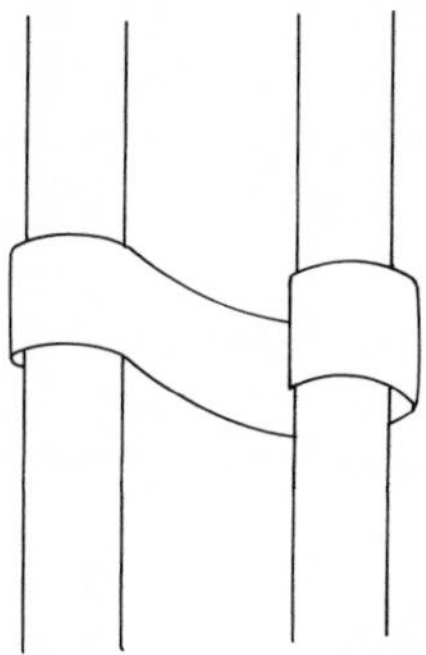

Fig. 2-7. Heister's lock. *(Adapted from Das: Obstetric Forceps, St. Louis, 1929, The C. V. Mosby Company.)*

The Chamberlen forceps possessed a rivet to unite the branches. When the forceps was used, however, a thong or binding was wrapped about the shanks and handles. Palfyn's parallel spoons also required a cloth binding about the handles to hold them together. Heister attempted to improve the function of Palfyn's instrument by uniting the shanks. He did this with an S-shaped metal strip which looped over one shank and beneath the other (Fig. 2-7). Although he admitted that this modification was not efficient, he emphasized the importance of uniting the branches with a mobile axis in order to avoid slippage of the blades. Unaware of other efforts, Dusée and Chapman in the 1730's were developing the locking mechanisms of their forceps which were to become the prototypes of the French and English schools.

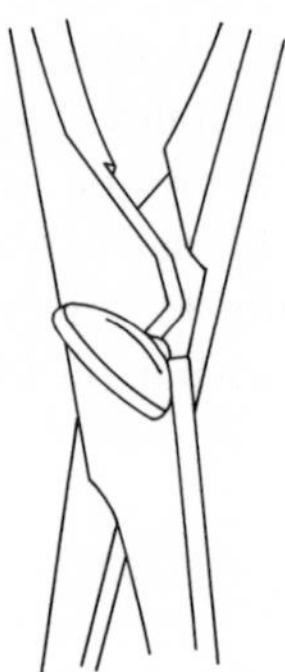

Fig. 2-8. French lock.

The French Lock

Dusée must be given the credit for the first successful attempt at articulating the branches of the obstetric forceps. He accomplished this by first flattening the shanks so that he could cross the blades in apposition to each other, and then joining the shanks by passing a screw through them.

Subsequent modifications utilizing either a detachable or semi-fixed screw or an upright button about which the opposing branch can rotate have become known as French locks (Fig. 2-8).

The English Lock

Chapman, Dusée's English contemporary, had made a pair of forceps whose branches each contained a mortise which allowed them to be fixed together. Originally it possessed a screw for fixation. By accident he lost the screw to his instrument and much to his surprise found that his forceps functioned better without absolute fixation of its branches.

Smellie, who simultaneously but independently of Levret and Pugh introduced the pelvic curve to obstetric forceps, must receive credit for the development of the English lock. It is ingeniously simple, consisting of a deep notch in each shank. When the shanks are crossed and in apposition, the shoulders of one notch oppose the shoulders of the other, thus keeping the instrument engaged. This type of lock is employed on the Simpson and Elliott forceps and their modifications (Fig. 2-9).

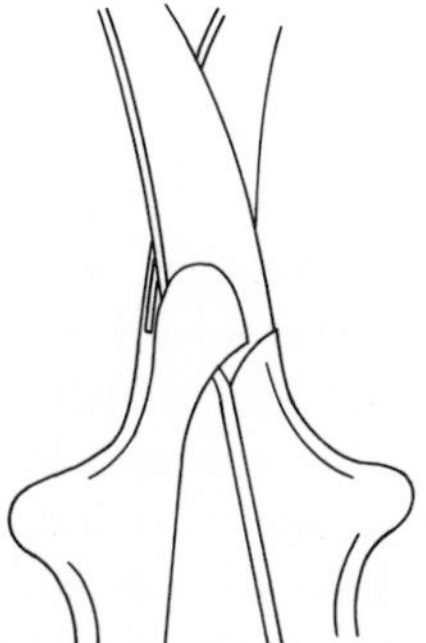

Fig. 2-9. English lock.

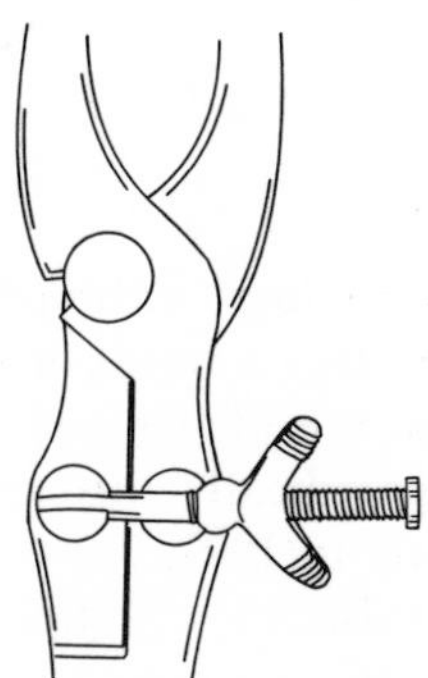

Fig. 2-10. German lock.

The German Lock

The locking mechanism of the forceps designed by the German school is the most rigid. It is a combination of a French or English lock at the shanks with an additional lock across the handles—a wing nut and screw. When the screw is snapped into place and the wing nut tightened down, the branches of the instrument become rigid. This forceful locking mechanism was to add security to the grasp of the blades on the fetal head (Fig. 2-10).

The Sliding Lock

The sliding lock which has become so popular in the past fifty years was introduced by Kielland. Barton also used this articulating mechanism. The lock is simple. About midway on the left shank is a raised L-shaped clamp. The right shank slides over the left and under the lip of the clamp. The mobility of the shanks permits the blades to adapt to an asynclytic head (Fig. 2-11).

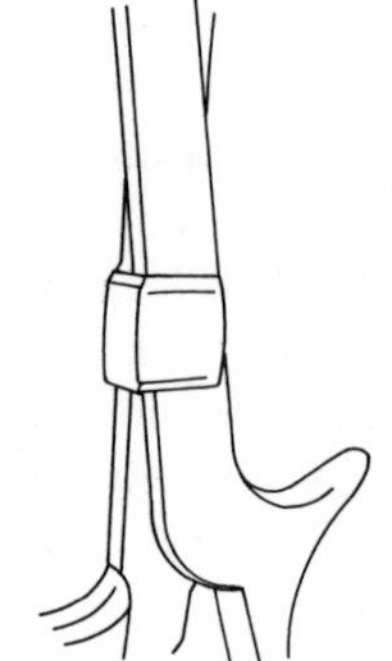

Fig. 2-11. Sliding lock.

The Pivot Lock

The pivot lock, although not commonly employed, warrants consideration. It is a result of the attempts of numerous forceps designers to uncross the blades and reduce compression. Such instruments appeared sporadically throughout the nineteenth century. It remained for Boerma in 1907, however, to perfect this lock. The locking mechanism consists of a protected axle at the base of one shank which rotates within a groove at the base of the opposite shank. The pivoting action of the lock allows the blades to open or close in an arc. In place

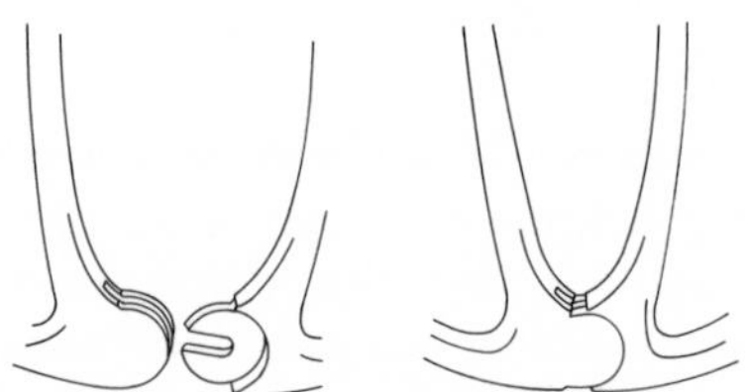

Fig. 2-12. Pivot lock, disengaged (*left*) and closed (*right*).

of a handle, there are simple finger guides. The author has used this type of locking mechanism and abbreviated handles in both an outlet and the modified Piper forceps (Fig. 2-12).[56,57]

HANDLES

The handles of the early obstetric forceps told an interesting story. Many terminated in hooks, perforators, or crotchets whose presence allowed the accoucheur to dismember the fetus if he could not extract it with the forceps. A strange but familiar paradox—one end to save a life, the other to destroy it. Some practitioners emphasized the destructive portion of their instrument; others, such as Freke, concealed the crotchet or hook beneath a flap in the handle.

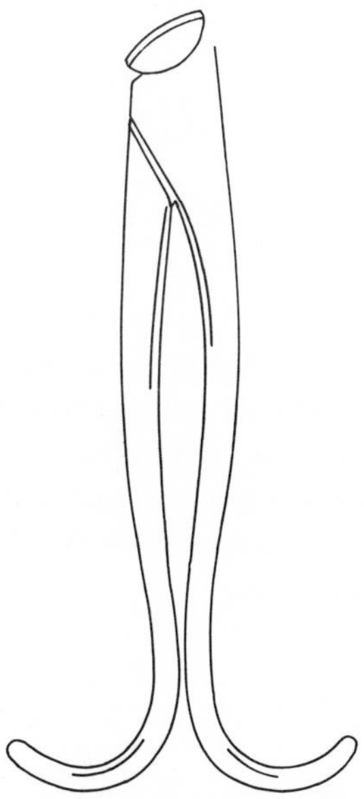

Fig. 2-13. Handles of early forceps.

A simple but important modification in forceps handles was that added by Johann Busch. Most handles until 1798 terminated in finger grips or rests which flared outward (Fig. 2-13). Busch moved these finger grips to the upper end of the handles beneath the lock, and there they have remained. Boerma, to augment his pivot lock, retained Busch's finger grips but eliminated the lower portion of the handles. Elliott added an adjustable transverse pin to the base of his handles to control compression (Fig. 2-14).

The handles of most modern forceps are similar. Most are hollow, while many have indented sides to enhance the grip. The handles of the Kielland vary in that they are solid, quite narrow, and separated.

The most significant change in the handles was made to accommodate the principle of axis-traction. Tarnier attached a traction bar beneath the handles and fastened it by wires to the heels of the blades.

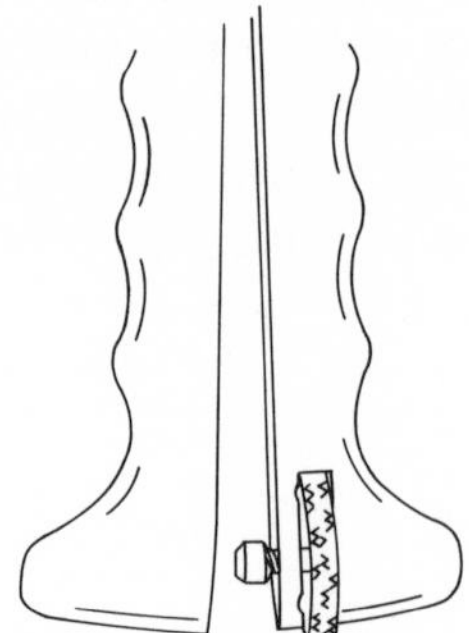

Fig. 2-14. Handles of Elliott forceps.

This enabled traction to be made in a plane continuous with the central pelvic curve. A directional marker indicated the angle of traction. Various modifications developed to suit other instruments, such as the Barton. The ultimate refinement, however, was the detachable traction handle of Bill,[9] which can be used with almost any conventional forceps (Fig. 2-15).

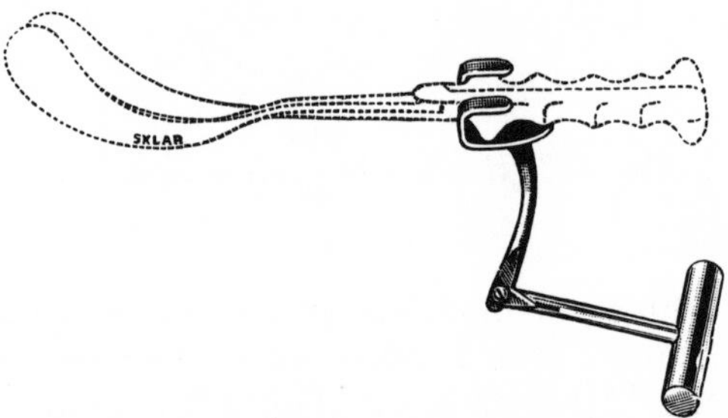

Fig. 2-15. Bill axis-traction handle. *(Courtesy of J. Sklar Manufacturing Company.)*

There have been numerous attempts to change the components of modern obstetric forceps. Among the most common alterations are: abbreviation of the handles; alterations of the lock; uncrossing the branches; and utilization of hinged symmetrical blades. Some of the more unique instruments include the spatulas of Thierry, the parallel forceps of Shute, and a well-engineered, complex instrument introduced by Miseo which employs a split universal joint. Other innovations have been introduced by Jacobs, LaBreck, and Mann. None of these forceps, however, has been subjected to adequate clinical evaluation to determine its proper place among the currently employed instruments.

Chapter Three

Functions of Obstetric Forceps

The functions of obstetric forceps are simple; the factors involved in accomplishing them—complex. There are only two functions which forceps should perform—traction and rotation. These can be performed independently or concurrently. In order for traction and rotation to be accomplished, however, a third function—compression—simultaneously occurs. Unfortunately, this factor is undesirable. It is what spurs the continuing seach for the ideal obstetric forceps: one that applies effective traction with minimal or safe compression.

There is a surprising paucity of recorded information regarding these factors, although it is more than one hundred years since Kristeller introduced his metric forceps. Kristeller's instrument was capable of measuring only the force of traction, but it represented the first attempt to quantitate the forces involved in the use of obstetric forceps. During the nineteenth century, numerous attempts were made to devise forceps with pulleys, cranks, and controls. Most were fearsome looking, but none so elaborate as that introduced by Jacobson of New York in 1905. His instrument, a traction apparatus which was to substitute mechanical exactness for human fallibility, was a fantastic device. It included a dial dynamometer, cross and traction bars, clamps, worm and gear, all of which finally terminated in a rotary hand wheel. It was so cumbersome and complex it never became more than a curiosity (Fig. 3-1).

In 1935 Wylie[113] evaluated the force of traction in 880 deliveries.

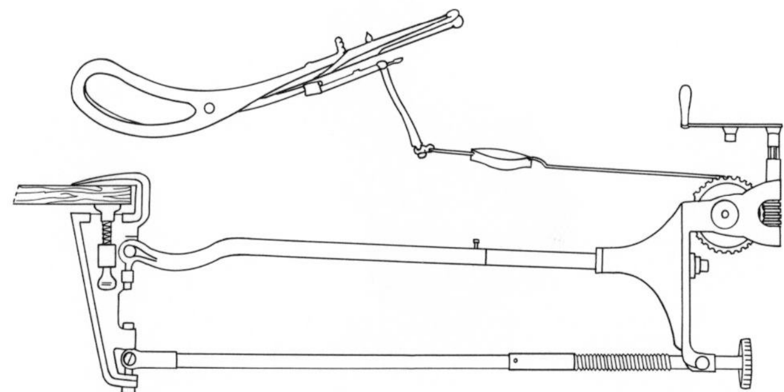

Fig. 3-1. Jacobson's forceps. *(Adapted from Das: Obstetric Forceps, St. Louis, 1929, The C. V. Mosby Company.)*

He used a spring gauge on a Bill axis-traction handle attached to a Tucker-McLane forceps. Wylie quantitatively confirmed the increased force required to deliver primiparas. Despite this significant contribution, another twenty-year hiatus occurred. Although the leading clinicians and teachers of this era preached conservatism and spoke of the forceps as compressive levers, no efforts were made to evaluate the forces involved. During the past decade, however, renewed impetus has come through the efforts of Fleming, Pearse,[73] Wylie,[114] Ullery and their co-workers as well as others.

The major factors which influence forceps performance are not well appreciated. They are: (*1*) the structure of the instrument; (*2*) the fetal head which the forceps must grasp; (*3*) the resistance of the maternal tissues; and (*4*) the force applied by the attendant. Each of these factors is dependent upon a multiplicity of smaller ones. Evaluation of problems involved requires special instrumentation, but it must be accomplished if obstetric forceps are to be understood and properly used.

COMPRESSION

The conventional obstetric forceps generate compression because they are levers of the first class. The handles are the lever arm of the applied force; the lock the fulcrum; and the shanks and blades the lever arm of the load (Fig. 3-2). Compression by the blades, therefore, is a direct function of the squeezing force applied at the handles. Instruments whose fixed locks are the fulcrum invite this force, whereas sliding and pivot locks require no compression of the handles to insure articulation of the branches. Some degree of compression, however, is a necessary accomplice to traction or rotation if slippage of the blades

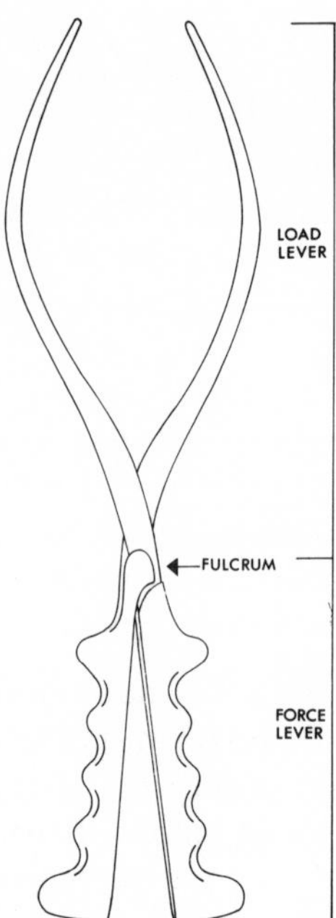

Fig. 3-2. Mechanics of conventional forceps.

is to be avoided. In a proper forceps application, the compressive force is distributed over the entire contour of the blades. If an inappropriate instrument is selected or poor application is made, pressure points can be created. These usually occur at the toes of the blades. The resultant indentations of the soft tissues of the fetal head, although usually temporary, are testimony to a poor choice of instrument or undue force.

The factors related to the fetus are the compressibility of the soft tissues and the ability of the cranial bones to overlap. The latter is influenced by the amount of molding which has occurred because of the forces of labor and the resistance of the maternal tissues. The size of the fetal head and its relationship to the capacity of the maternal pelvis also have bearing on the amount of traction required and the accompanying compression.

Fleming, Brandeberry, and Pearse have developed an ingenious metric forceps to measure compressive force. Their instrument has permanent strain gauges fixed in the shank of the left branch which connect to a twin channel recorder and amplifier. Each delivery can be recorded on continually moving paper and the record is called an electro-delivery-gram (EDG). These workers acknowledge that the total compressive force is due to the pressure applied at the handles, the resistance of the fetal head, and the resistance or lack thereof of the maternal tissues. The maximum compressive force recorded was 5.5 lb. in a limited series of cases. Their data has been confirmed by Ullery and his associates and by Pearse.[73] The latter's series is the largest studied by this technic. Pearse found the average maximum compression of one blade is 4.95 lb. and the total compressive force (average maximum force × seconds held) is 152 lb. He also concludes that "compression was not directly proportional to traction, was usually quite constant after application, and varied with traction primarily in premature infants and those in the occipitoposterior position."

Kelly and Sines have recently performed more elaborate studies to assess the compression and traction forces of obstetric forceps. They implanted 16 strain gauges along the shank and blade of a Simpson forceps. From a limited series of deliveries, they conclude that "the peak or maximal force is probably the most important factor."

To minimize the compressive force of obstetric forceps, the author has designed a pair of outlet forceps based on the principle of divergence. By this design, the instrument is converted from a first-class to a third-class lever. The physical factor of compression for the author's divergent forceps and for a conventional crossed forceps (Simpson) was analyzed by free-body diagrams. These studies were performed by the Columbus, Ohio laboratories of the Battelle Memorial Institute. (The Institute also designed and produced the instrumentation for the studies of Fleming, Pearse, and Ullery.)

A free-body diagram is a method used to analyze the action of forces on a given body. The body is isolated by removing all contacting and attached bodies and replacing them by vectors representing the forces which they exert on the isolated body. Thus a free-body diagram is created, and to provide static equilibrium, the vector sum of these forces and their moments must equal zero. The forces studied were as follows:

F_t = force applied on traction handle
F_s = force applied (clamping force) by forceps spoons (blades)
F_h = tractive force applied to Simpson forceps by traction handle
F_c = clamping force applied to Simpson handles

Equations were then developed using free-body diagrams for defining F_s, the clamping or compressive force applied through the blades, in terms of F_t and F_c. It should be pointed out that the coefficients in both equations are entirely dependent on the geometry of the forceps and assumed lines of force-vector action.

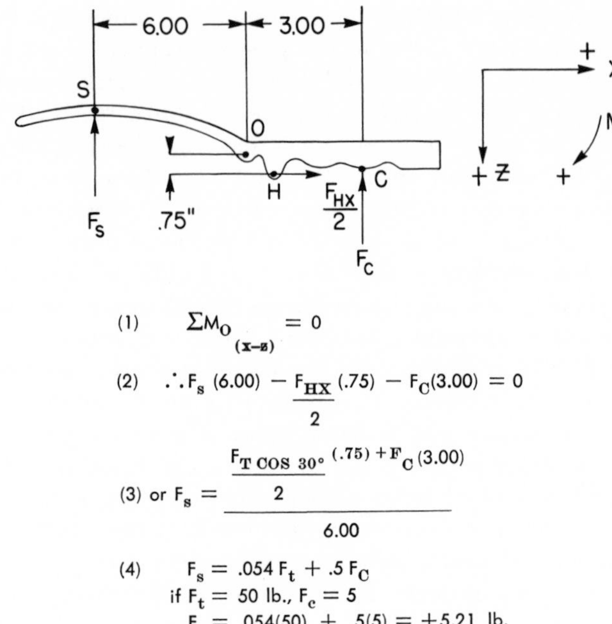

Fig. 3-3. Free-body diagram of crossed forceps branch. *(From Laufe, L. E. Amer. J. Obstet. Gynec. 101:509, 1968.)*

$$F_s \text{ for Simpson model} = 0.054\ (F_t) + 0.5\ (F_c)$$
$$F_s \text{ for Divergent model} = 0.053\ (F_t)$$

Using the above equations and setting $F_t = 50$ lb. for both models and $F_c = 5$ lb. for the Simpson model, the crossed forceps exerts a positive force of 5.21 lb. on the fetal head (Fig. 3-3). The divergent forceps exerts a negative force of 2.64 lb. (Fig. 3-4). Positive force with the latter instrument is exerted on the pelvic walls.

The divergent forceps is incapable of producing compression of the fetal head unless the *shanks* are squeezed. It should function as an interface between the fetal head and pelvic walls. Although theoretically sound, the instrument remains to be clinically proven.

TRACTION

More data is available on the force of traction than on compressive force, but the related factors are more difficult to assess. Interestingly enough, Kristeller's figure of 35 lb. of average traction force is in keeping with the data of recent investigators. Wylie[114] and Mishell and Kelly used a spring gauge in a Bill axis-traction handle, which Wiley later named "axis tractionometer." He recorded an average pull

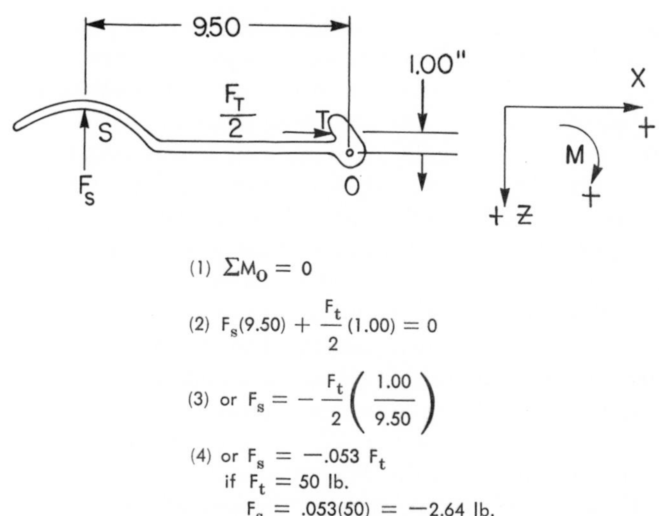

Fig. 3-4. Free-body diagram of divergent forceps branch. (*From Laufe, L. E. Amer. J. Obstet. Gynec. 101:509, 1968.*)

or peak force of 12.4 kg. Wylie commented on the extreme variations encountered between individual cases and concluded that the risk of injury to the fetus is negligible if the force is under 20 kg.

Fleming, Pearse,[73] Ullery and their respective co-workers employed a different technic. Using electronic strain gauges attached to a Bill axis-traction handle, Ullery's group recorded an average maximum force with each individual traction of 18 kg. for a primipara and 13 kg. for a multipara. The average total force applied to the fetal head in the primipara was over 900 kg. in 65 sec. and in the multipara, 727 kg. during an 83-sec. interval. Pearse carried out similar studies on a larger group of patients and concluded the total forces were best visualized by computing the time-force area as well as recording the single maximum point. He found traction forces elevated in deliveries of first and second infants, occiput-posterior positions, and infants weighing over 3,000 gm. These investigators have correlated the fetal heart rate as an index of fetal response. Fetal bradycardia was noted in all cases of forceps traction, but did not appreciably differ from that noted in spontaneous deliveries. Most investigators have concluded that similar amounts of force are generated in spontaneous deliveries.

To fully comprehend the accomplishment of a forceps delivery, we must appreciate Newton's Second Law of Motion. This fundamental law of mechanics states that when a body is acted upon by a constant force, its resulting acceleration will be in the direction of the applied force and is proportional to the force and inversely proportional to the mass. Thus the rapidity with which a delivery will be accomplished can be a direct function of the force applied as well as decreased resistance. To further appreciate force, one must remember that it involves all three of the fundatmental units of mechanics: length, mass, and time. Obstetrically speaking, this means that the force applied in forceps traction depends upon: how big the baby; how far we move it; and in what period of time. More important is the factor of jerking. "Jerk" means the time-rate of change of acceleration. In other words, a sudden change in the rate of acceleration is probably more hazardous to the fetus than the total force of traction.

The obstetric factors which contribute to the total force of traction employed with forceps include the resistance of the passage (maternal tissues) and the fetal head. Maternal resistance is a composite of soft-tissue resistance as well as that of the bony pelvis. The soft-tissue resistance is a function of the density, elasticity, and thickness of the tissues. These factors in turn vary with the patient's age, height, weight, and parity. They are well exemplified by the reduced resistance offered by the multiparous patient and the lessening of resistance accomplished with episiotomy. The bony resistance is a function of the type of pelvis and its relationship to the size of the baby.

The size of the fetal head also influences the amount of resistance to traction. Assuming that normal fetal heads are of the same density, then it is logical that the mass will be proportionate to the volume. The larger the head, the greater the force required for extraction. Another related factor is the attitude or position of the head, since some diameters are more favorable than others for easy extraction. Whether or not the fetus can actively resist the force of traction has yet to be proven.

An additional and probably the most important physical factor which contributes to the total force of traction is friction. The coefficient of friction between the fetal head and forceps is low, and most applications are firm to insure a secure grasp of the fetal head. The forceps also must work against the static friction of the maternal soft tissues. This factor, of course, is also present in spontaneous deliveries. With forceps it is altered by the type of force applied, since starting friction is greater than kinetic friction. All too familiar is the soft-tissue trauma which can ensue when traction is injudiciously initiated.

ROTATION

Smellie in 1752 was the first to record the use of the obstetric forceps as a rotator. More than one hundred years later, in 1853, Scanzoni developed and reported his forceps operation of instrumental rotation. The actual principles by which forceps can serve to correct the position of the head in the pelvis were finally clarified by Tarnier in 1881. In attempting to allow the fetal head freedom of rotary movement through the pelvis, he demonstrated the rotary action of conventional forceps. When the handles are twisted, the toes of the blades will describe an arc because of their pelvic curve. To accomplish rotation about an axis, it is necessary for the handles to describe a wide arc outside the pelvis. With this maneuver the toes of the blades become the central point of rotation (Fig. 3-5).

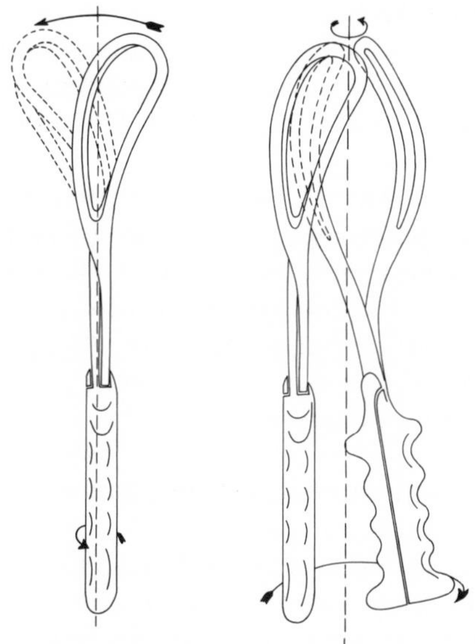

Fig. 3-5. Rotation of forceps.

The radius of the arc which the handles of obstetric forceps must transcribe for successful rotation is related to the pelvic curve which the blade possesses. For conventional instruments with a full pelvic curve, the rotary arc of the handles must be wide. As the functional pelvic curve of the blades is reduced, the arc diminishes. This is best exemplified by the Kielland forceps, in which the pelvic curve is reversed by the angulation of the shanks. With this instrument, efficient and successful rotation is accomplished by merely imparting a twisting motion to the handles. Special forceps for rotation have been designed to capitalize on this motion.

When obstetric forceps are used as rotators, most of the mechanical factors of traction and compression remain. Some are altered. Instrumental rotation of the fetal head is dependent upon the construction of the forceps; the mass to be rotated; the resistance of the maternal tissues; and the force applied.

As with traction, increased mass of the fetal head requires increased force for rotation. The relationship of the size of the head to the spaciousness of the pelvis also influences the ease of forceps rotation. For this reason, Bill[8,10] advocated elevation of the head to a higher, more spacious pelvic plane prior to rotation. A well-molded head which seems tightly wedged into the pelvis frequently rotates with ease once it has been elevated. How much the fetus actively resists forced rotation is unknown.

Although perineal resistance is not a factor in midpelvic rotations, soft-tissue resistance is still present and dependent on such factors as multiparity, elasticity, and friction. A well-contracted uterus adds resistance to rotary fetal motion.

Since all of these factors as well as the laws of acceleration and deceleration are integral components of forceps rotation, the rate at which any rotary maneuver is performed is of cardinal importance. Rotation must be initiated and performed with proper gentle technic if compression is to be kept at a minimum. Advantage will then be taken of the ability of the maternal tissues to alter their resistance and of the fetus to alter its position.

NATURAL FORCES OF DELIVERY

Before definitive conclusions can be drawn from the foregoing data regarding the forces generated in forceps deliveries, comparisons must be made with the forces involved in spontaneous deliveries. During labor and spontaneous delivery other factors come into action. These are the contractile force of the uterus and the expulsive efforts of the abdominal wall. The pioneers who have measured the behavior of the uterus during labor and delivery are few. Using clever devices such as tokodynanometers, intrauterine receptors, and intramyometrical balloons, Reynolds,[82-84] Karlson, Caldeyro-Barcia[13-14] and others have made significant contributions to our understanding of the forces of labor and delivery. Extrapolating their data, Pearse[74] calculates the downward force of the uterine contraction as being approximately 4.2 kg. and concludes that it would be doubled with the expulsive effort of bearing down.

Maternal soft- and bony-tissue resistance occurs in spontaneous deliveries, of course, as does the ability of the fetal head to adapt to the contour of the birth canal. The same factors of multiparity, tissue elasticity, and friction also exist. These forces, as well as the resistance offered by the effacing and dilating cervix, all contribute to the pressures to which the fetal head is subjected. Unfortunately, adequate data regarding these forces is not yet available. Although the technical problems involved in obtaining this data are formidable, some of it should be within reach.

How much of the total natural forces of the second stage of labor the fetal head is spared by a judicious forceps delivery is unknown. Most agree, however, on the concept of prophylactic outlet forceps as a procedure which limits the total cumulative force and pressure the fetal head must undergo.

Although data is accumulating regarding the individual forces of compression, traction, and rotation generated by obstetric forceps, it is a meager beginning. The total resultant force of these component functions has not been evaluated. How much traction or rotation augments compression must be investigated and compared to the natural forces of labor. This appears to be a most neglected but fertile field of clinical investigation. Until better information on the forces of spontaneous delivery is available, the recorded documentation available on forceps traction and compression cannot be used as a standard. No comparison exists.

All of the components which contribute to the function of obstetric forceps are interdependent and occur either simultaneously or sequentially. One aspect cannot be separated from another. The obstetrician must fully appreciate each phase of the delivery: the instrument, the object, the resistance, and the force applied. His knowledge of the pelvis; ability to assess a problem; comprehension of the advantages and limitations of various instruments; and his ability to properly use these tools are the ultimate factors in the conduct of a forceps delivery.

Chapter Four

Conventional Obstetric Forceps

✻

CLASSIC FORCEPS

There are two classic obstetric forceps: the Simpson and the Elliott. They have been the progenitors of more offspring than any other forceps during the past century. These instruments and their variations perform the majority of the forceps deliveries in this country. They retain and merit extensive popularity. Some obstetricians, however, have adopted one type to the exclusion of the other. This is unfortunate, for each forceps has its advantages. They should be considered as complementary rather than as competitive instruments.

Simpson Forceps

The classic or long Simpson forceps has an overall length of 35 cm. (*see* Fig. 1-6). More than one-half of the instrument (18 cm.) is devoted to the gradually tapered, fenestrated blades. This provides for a shallow cephalic curve which allows excellent application of the blades to large and well-molded heads. The short parallel shanks diverge rapidly from the English lock and handle. Simpson emphasized traction rather than compression and advocated inserting a finger between the shanks as a cushioning effect. The parallel shanks do have a slight disadvantage, however, in that they can markedly distend the perineum.

A most popular variation of the Simpson forceps is that of DeLee.[24] He lengthened the shanks, enlarged the finger grips, and modified the handles (Fig. 4-1). The DeLee forceps is available in short and long models. The Simpson forceps has also served as the prototype for

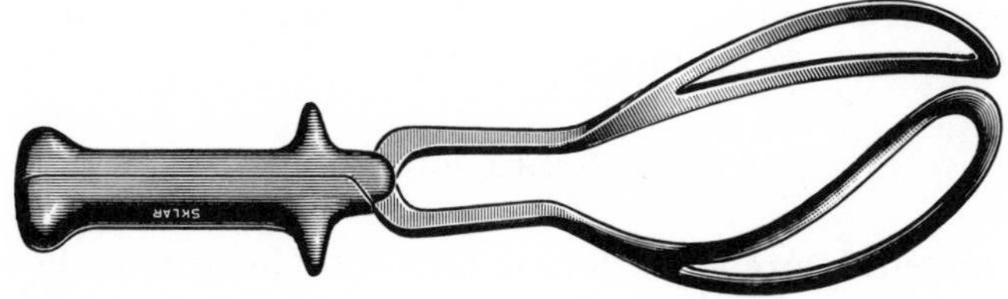

Fig. 4-1. DeLee forceps. *(Courtesy of J. Sklar Manufacturing Company.)*

numerous axis-traction forceps. The Hawks-Dennen forceps is a relatively recent adaptation employing the principle of fixed axis-traction.

Elliott Forceps

The short forceps introduced by Elliott of New York differs from the Simpson in its blades, shanks, and handles. The blades are shorter (15 cm.). Their cephalic curve is more accentuated and therefore more suitable for an average-sized fetal head or one which has not undergone extensive molding. When they are applied to a large head, the toes of the blades tend to produce preauricular pressure points. The shanks of the Elliott forceps are overlapping and hence do not distend the perineum as do those of the Simpson. The original Elliott forceps has an adjustable screw and pin at the base of the right handle to regulate lateral pressure (*see* Fig. 1-7).

The Elliott forceps is available as both long (38 cm.) and short (32 cm.) models. The long Elliott forceps has blades which are identical in length to the Simpson (18 cm.). Their accentuated cephalic curve is partially retained, however. When the branches of the long Elliott forceps are articulated and approximated, the toes of the blades are 2.5 cm. apart. The toes of the Simpson blades are 3.5 cm. apart and the toes of the blades of the short Elliott forceps are 1.5 cm. apart.

There are numerous modifications of the Elliott instrument but the most popular is the Tucker-McLane. It is available with either solid or semisolid (Luikart) blades. This and the fenestrated Bailey-William-

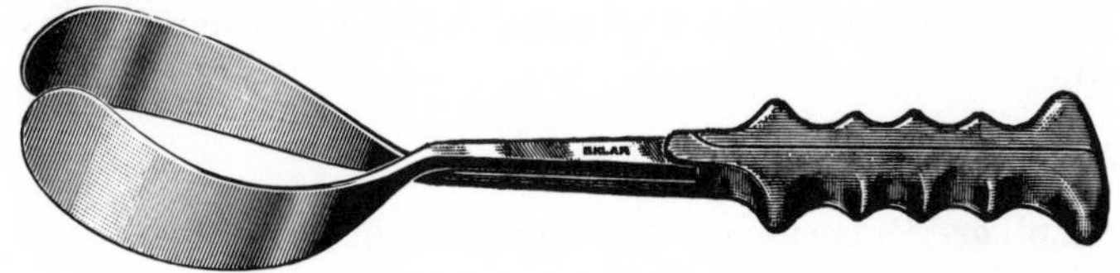

Fig. 4-2. Tucker-McLane forceps. *(Courtesy of J. Sklar Manufacturing Company.)*

son forceps have lengthened shanks which result in an accentuation of the cephalic curve of the blades (Fig. 4-2).

RECENT INNOVATIONS

Four obstetric forceps which have been introduced recently warrant consideration here. They are the Hawks-Dennen,[25] Luikart,[59] Shute, and the author's outlet forceps.[57] The first two are improved modifications of accepted principles of forceps design. The Shute forceps is a modern adaptation of the parallel principle. The author's forceps is a simple outlet instrument based on the principle of divergence in order to capitalize on the function of third-class levers.

Hawks-Dennen Forceps

In 1931 Dr. Edward Dennen presented before the New York Obstetrical Society the forceps he and Dr. W. M. Hawks had designed.[25] Their purpose was to construct a simple, light, fixed axis-traction forceps (Fig. 4-3). The blades of their instrument are a modification of the Simpson. The tips or toes are slightly lengthened, the curve of the posterior lips is exaggerated, and the inner surface is beveled like the Kielland. The parallel shanks are bent to form a perineal curve.

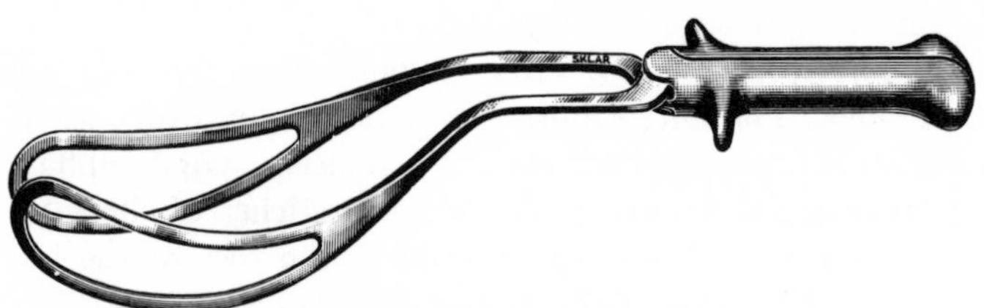

Fig. 4-3. Hawks-Dennen forceps. *(Courtesy of J. Sklar Manufacturing Company.)*

The instrument has a traditional English lock and handles. The backward bend of the proximal shanks and handles provides the fixed axis-traction.

Luikart Forceps

The Luikart[59] instrument includes some of the best features of the most popular instruments. Luikart's purpose was to add increased safety to his forceps. The forceps can be described as a Tucker-McLane with three basic modifications. (*1*) The shanks are overlapping and

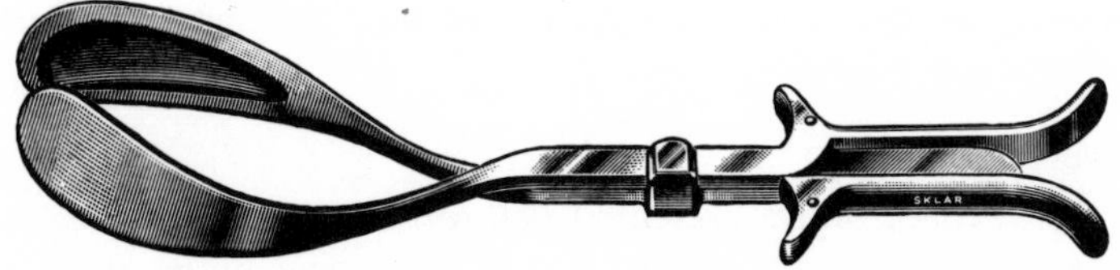

Fig. 4-4. Luikart forceps. *(Courtesy of J. Sklar Manufacturing Company.)*

have a sliding lock. (*2*) The handles are an adaptation of the Kielland. The left one has a flat extension which expands medially to fill the gap between them. Luikart's intention was to reduce the danger of excessive pressure being applied. (*3*) The blades have the same contour as the Tucker-McLane but with a depression on the cephalic side, producing a pseudofenestration. This modification has achieved widespread popularity and has been applied to many other forceps (Fig. 4-4).

Luikart also modified the Bill axis-traction handle so that it would

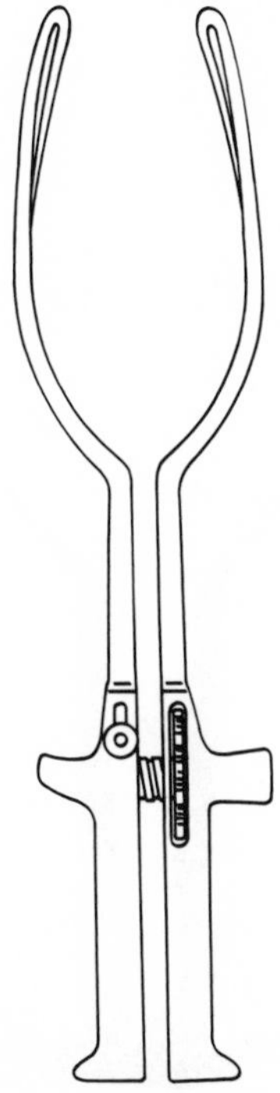

Fig. 4-5. Shute forceps.

fit, not over the lock and finger grips, but over the shanks of his forceps.

Shute Forceps

In 1958 Wallace Shute presented before the Chicago Gynecological Society a parallel forceps which he had been developing since 1941. Although he believed his instrument to be based on a new principle, in reality it is a modern adaptation of the parallel spoons of Palfyn (Fig. 4-5). The unique feature of the Shute forceps is the inclusion of a locking mechanism within the shanks and horn on the left shaft to provide perfect parallelism of the branches. It consists of a double-threaded screw which has a T-shaped bar fused to its free end. The screw is controlled by a large wheel which is housed in an axial slot in the left shank. The wheel regulates the distance at which the T-end of the screw will engage with the opposite shank. The mechanism is calibrated so that one full turn of the wheel moves the screw and the blades a distance of 4 mm.

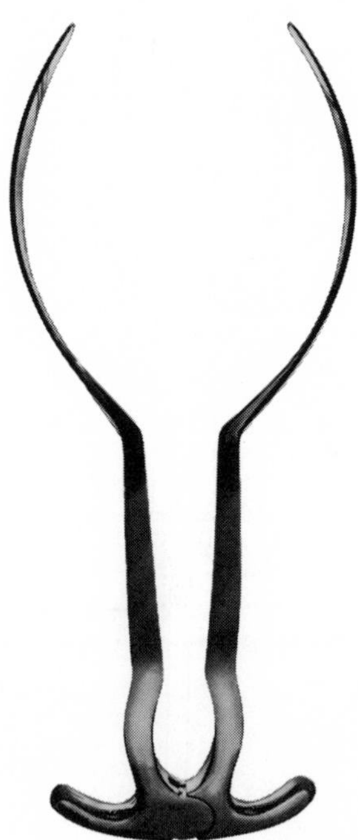

Fig. 4-6. Divergent outlet forceps, pivot lock engaged. *(From Laufe, L. E. Amer. J. Obstet. Gynec. 101:509, 1968.)*

The blades of the Shute forceps are slightly shorter than the Simpson and have a shallower cephalic curve to avoid undue pressure points. Shute also elongated the shanks in order to use the instrument for mid-forceps applications and for the aftercoming head.

Pearse[75] has instrumented a Shute forceps with strain gauges to evaluate the compressive force. From a very limited series, he has yet to observe any significant difference between this instrument and the Simpson.

Divergent Forceps

The author[57] has designed a forceps for outlet vertex extractions based on the divergent principle of Thenance. The purpose of utilizing this principle is to convert the forceps into a third-class lever in order to reduce the compressive force applied to the fetal head. The branches do not cross but originate as a V from the pivot lock, which has lateral mobility. The forceps includes components of some of the most cur-

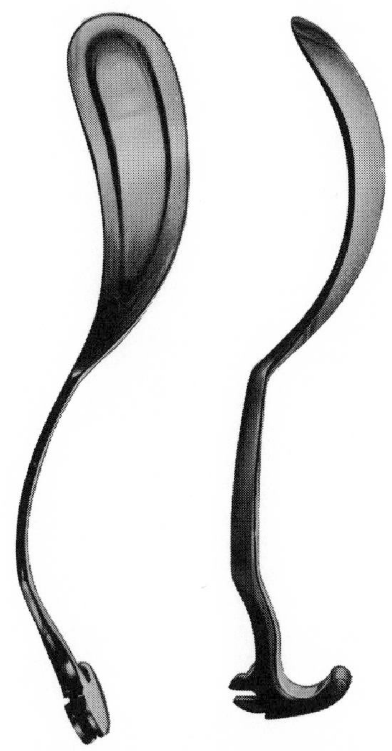

Fig. 4-7. Divergent outlet forceps, branches separated. *(From Laufe, L. E. Amer. J. Obstet. Gynec. 101:509, 1968.)*

rently popular instruments. It has an overall length of 31.5 cm. The blades, which are 15 cm. in length, have the contour of Elliott forceps with the Luikart modification. The shanks are parallel, 14 cm. in length, and have a perineal curve so that the axis-traction principle is inherent in the use of the forceps (Figs. 4-6 and 4-7).

When the instrument is closed, the shanks are adjacent but will diverge from the pivot lock to allow the blades to fit any sized head. The shanks separate as they approach the pivot lock so that when used, they allow the admission of the middle finger of the attendant to provide a cushioning effect and to inhibit compression. The instrument terminates in lateral finger grips rather than traditional handles. The locks and grips are identical to the ones used on the short Piper forceps.

The essential features of this instrument consist of Elliott blades with Luikart modification, a perineal curve in the shank, and a pivot lock with finger grips.

*

Chapter Five

*

Special Obstetric Instruments

*

Deliveries which demand special obstetric instruments can be classified as: (*1*) those requiring instrumental rotation; (*2*) those requiring increased traction; and (*3*) breech deliveries requiring management of an aftercoming head. The majority of the instruments which have been designed for these problems are relatively recent additions to the obstetrician's armamentarium. New instruments as well as modifications of accepted ones continue to evolve for the management of these complications, but only a few have achieved acceptance. It behooves the clinician, however, not only to be familiar with the special forceps in common use, but to be sensitive to the potential value of each new one.

FORCEPS FOR ARRESTS OF ROTATION

Although any conventional forceps can be used for rotation, there are special instruments with unique advantages for the management of rotary arrests. They were designed for specific purposes and have structural modifications which enhance their function as rotators. Some are also modified to accommodate their application to the arrested fetal head.

The most commonly employed special obstetric forceps for the management of occiput transverse or posterior arrests is the Kielland. The Barton forceps, although primarily a tractor, is included here since it also was designed for the management of certain transverse arrests. Its unique ability is the delivery of a transverse arrest as a transverse. The Kielland-Barton (K-B) forceps, an instrument designed by the author,[54,55] combines the advantages of the Barton application with the rotary ability of the Kielland instrument. Other instruments are available and continue to appear for the management of the problem. Although well designed, many are extremely complex, employing numerous moving parts which limits their production, distribution, and perhaps their acceptance.

Kielland Forceps

In 1915 Christian Kielland of Norway introduced a forceps which had considerable impact upon the obstetric world. The concept of a functional pelvic curve had become so well implanted in the minds of most clinicians that Kielland's instrument, which negated the pelvic curve, appeared as a radical departure. Closer scrutiny, however, revealed it to be a well-designed and -engineered instrument capable of performing Kielland's objective: a biparietal forceps application to the fetal head in any pelvic diameter.

Kielland's intent was to capitalize on the triangular space in the lower uterine segment between the shoulder and fetal head. He utilized this space for the insertion, rotation, and application of the anterior branch to transverse positions. To accomplish this and subsequent rotation, he counteracted the pelvic curve by altering the angulation of the blade with the shank; placed markers on the handles for orientation to the occiput; and introduced the sliding lock to compensate for asynclytism.

Enthusiasm for this instrument was quick to follow. Unfortunately, in many instances proper technical discipline was disregarded. During the next decade numerous reports from the Continent indicted the instrument as causing perforation of the lower uterine segment, interruption of placental implantation, and even laceration of the umbilical cord.

Fortunately, others were able to appreciate Kielland's motives. Proper utilization, and other technics of application, confirmed Kielland's objectives and principles of design. Today this instrument is probably the most popular rotator of all obstetric forceps and has become one of the most valuable instruments in modern operative obstetrics.

Construction

The Kielland forceps has an overall length of 40 cm. proportioned as follows: handles, 12 cm.; shanks, 13 cm.; and blades, 15 cm. The handles are narrow, solid, and separated. Their lateral finger grips possess elevated buttons which serve as directional markers for orientation to the occiput. The shanks are overlapping and they articulate by a sliding lock. The classic instrument has fenestrated blades 15 cm. in length and 4 cm. in breadth, slightly thicker than most others because of their rounded or beveled inner surface. The blades diverge rapidly from the shanks, enlarging the posterior component of the cephalic curve. They are capable of fitting a large and extensively molded head.

When viewed laterally, the Kielland forceps has a straight or bayonet appearance (*see* Fig. 1-8). This is because the superior aspect of the instrument follows a horizontal line. When held in this plane, the inferior aspect of the blades dips beneath the horizontal, reversing the pelvic curve.

Actually the contour of the blades is identical to the blades of an Elliott-type instrument, but they are oriented into a different plane by the angles at which they join the shanks (*see* Fig. 2-6). This offset angle is what negates the function of the pelvic curve when the forceps is used. The overall horizontal orientation of the instrument allows for the classic application and enhances its ability as a rotator. Some functional aspect of the pelvic curve can be restored, however, if the handles are appropriately dropped beneath the horizontal plane during traction.

Function

The primary function of the Kielland forceps is rotation. Its secondary function is traction, but only if the vertex is oriented to the anteroposterior pelvic plane.

The Barton Forceps

Of all the obstetric forceps in current use, the Barton instrument is the most unique. Easily recognized by the offset angulation of its blades and shanks, it has a limited but explicit function.

The instrument has an interesting history. It was designed by Lyman G. Barton, a most imaginative physician who practiced in Plattsburg, New York. His inventions were prolific and included such items as anesthetic containers and orthopedic tables as well as his obstetric forceps. Since Barton apparently attended numerous home deliveries in the Plattsburg area, one can speculate that he frequently observed multiparas with late uterine inertia. In most of these instances, the fetal head would be in the transverse diameter of the midpelvis or higher. He designed his instrument with the intent of making it capable of extracting the head in the transverse plane.

According to Bachman, who corresponded with Dr. Barton, the instrument had been conceived some twenty years prior to its formal introduction. The first model was rather crude, and those to whom

Barton showed it doubted its practicality but encouraged him regarding the theoretical aspects of the instrument. In 1924 he showed a refined drawing of his forceps to Dr. A. D. Campbell of Montreal, who advised him to proceed. The instrument was completed in October, 1924 and first used in December of that year. Two months later it was exhibited to the American Gynecological Club and finally presented to the New York Obstetrical Society in November, 1925.

Construction

The unique features of the Barton forceps are the hinged anterior blade and the angulation of the shanks with the blades. Instead of having right and left branches, this instrument is oriented to the anteroposterior planes of the pelvis. The hinged branch is the anterior one, the rigid branch the posterior. These features allow the pelvic and cephalic curve of the posterior blade to assume a parallel relationship when applied to a transverse head.

To fully comprehend the construction of the Barton forceps, it must be viewed from its posture of application (*see* Fig. 1-9). The handles, which are solid and measure 12 cm. in length, have a vertical rather than horizontal relationship to each other. They lead into parallel, adjacent shanks which are 11 cm. in length. The posterior branch has a sliding lock which allows the anterior branch to glide beside it. The fenestrated blades (15 cm. in length) are symmetrical, 5 cm. in breadth, and have a smooth cephalic surface. They join the shanks at a 50° angle. This is the normal angle between the axis of the pelvic inlet and outlet and allows the forceps to be applied in the anteroposterior diameter of the pelvis.

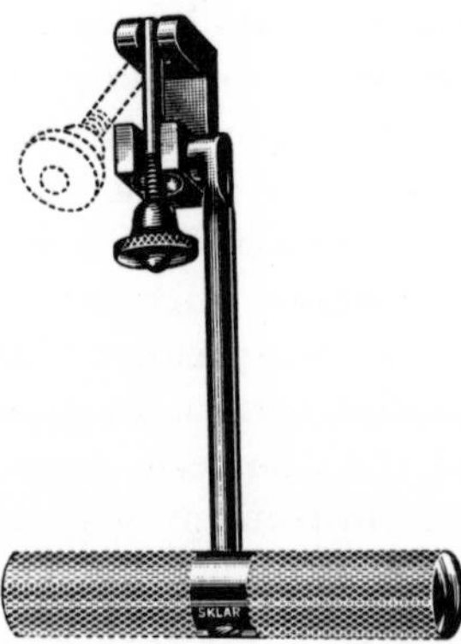

Fig. 5-1. Barton traction bar. *(Courtesy of J. Sklar Manufacturing Company.)*

In order to allow the anterior blade to be applied behind the symphysis for transverse arrests, it possesses a hinge. The hinge is located at the junction of the blade and shank and has a 50° arc of mobility. The posterior blade appears spoonlike in its symmetry and is unique in its adaptation to the pelvis. The hinged anterior blade and sliding lock allow the space between the blades to remain symmetrical, yet adaptable to heads of varying sizes.

Available with this instrument is an axis-traction bar that Barton designed. It attaches about the shanks near the handles and consists of a customary cross bar handle pivoted on the end of a traction rod (Fig. 5-1). If the forceps is used for rotation, with resulting lateral angulation of the shanks and handles, the traction bar can act as a compensatory means for applying traction in the central pelvic plane.

Function

The primary function of the Barton forceps is traction. This is limited to traction of a transverse fetal head in the transverse pelvic plane. The instrument can be used secondarily as a rotator in the management of occiput transverse and posterior positions. When so utilized, however, the ability of the forceps for traction becomes markedly reduced unless the traction bar is used, or traction is applied at the crotch of the blades.

The Kielland-Barton (K-B) Forceps

The Kielland-Barton (K-B) forceps is an attempt to combine the advantages of the Kielland and the Barton forceps while simultaneously overcoming their limitations. The instrument was designed for the management of occiput transverse and posterior positions. It is to be applied as the Barton instrument and utilized for rotation and extraction as the Kielland forceps. This instrument was introduced by the author in 1956[54] and refined in 1959.[55]

Construction

The K-B forceps is constructed on a Kielland frame but has the symmetrical blades of the Barton forceps. The unique feature of the instrument is the selective spring hinge located in the shank of one branch. The comparative construction data of these three instruments are summarized in Table 5-1.

At first glance the K-B forceps appears quite similar to the Kielland in its construction. Closer scrutiny of the instrument, however, reveals numerous mechanical variations. Although the proportions of blade, shank, and handle are identical to the Kielland, the overall weight is less because of the reduction in breadth and thickness of the com-

TABLE 5-I
COMPARATIVE DATA OF BARTON, KIELLAND, AND K-B FORCEPS

Length	Barton	Kielland	K-B
Handles	12 cm.	12 cm.	12 cm.
Shanks	11 cm.	13 cm.	13 cm.
Blades	15 cm.	15 cm.	15 cm.
Blade breadth	5 cm.	4 cm.	4 cm.
Blade shape	Symmetrical	Asymmetrical (conventional)	Symmetrical
Hinge	Present	Absent	Selective
Pelvic curve	Present	Present (nonfunctional)	Absent

ponents. The blades are 4 cm. in breadth. Their absolute symmetry eliminates the need for directional markers on the handles and reduces the functional pelvic curve to the minimum, since the blades extend only 2 cm. on either side of their median axis. The forceps is available either with fenestrated or solid blades (Luikart modification). (*See* Figs. 5-2 and 5-3.)

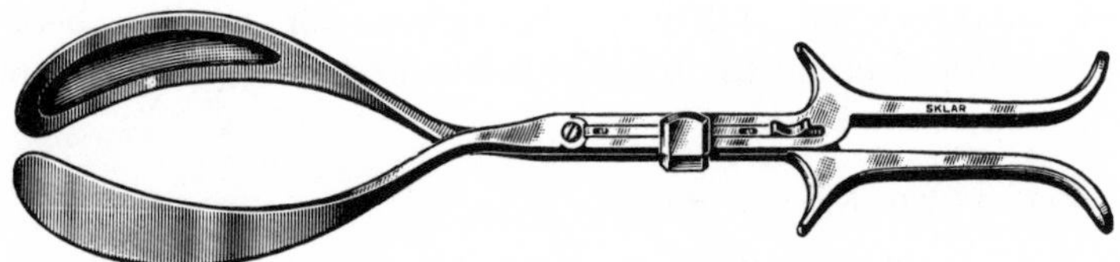

Fig. 5-2. Kielland-Barton forceps, Luikart modification. *(Courtesy of J. Sklar Manufacturing Company.)*

Located within the shank of one branch is a selective hinge. Its purpose is to allow this blade either to be rigid or flail (Fig. 5-3). The hinge is 5 cm. from the junction of the shank and blade, making the flail portion of the forceps 20 cm. in length. This distance assures that the hinge will be at or outside the vulvar orifice following application, thus avoiding possible trauma to the maternal soft tissues.

The locking mechanism of the selective hinge consists of a sliding member within the shank of the hinged blade. This sliding member runs the length of the shank and rests against a spring near the handle (Fig. 5-4). At the handle end of this member is a finger grip so that pressure may be applied against the spring behind it. When this is done, the lock is disengaged (Fig. 5-5). When no pressure is exerted, the spring is at rest and the distal end of the sliding member fits into a groove at the base of the blade (Fig. 5-4).

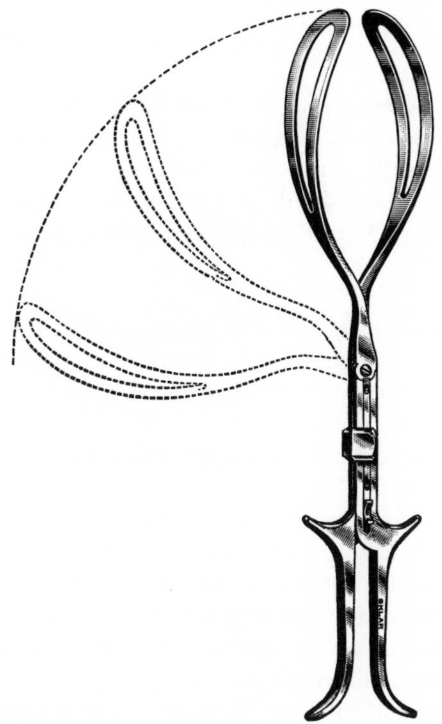

Fig. 5-3. Kielland-Barton forceps, hinged branch unlocked.
(Courtesy of J. Sklar Manufacturing Company.)

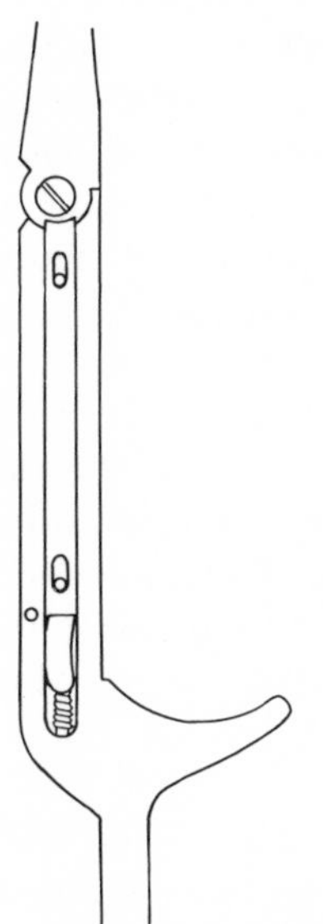

Fig. 5-4. Selective lock of Kielland-Barton forceps, engaged.

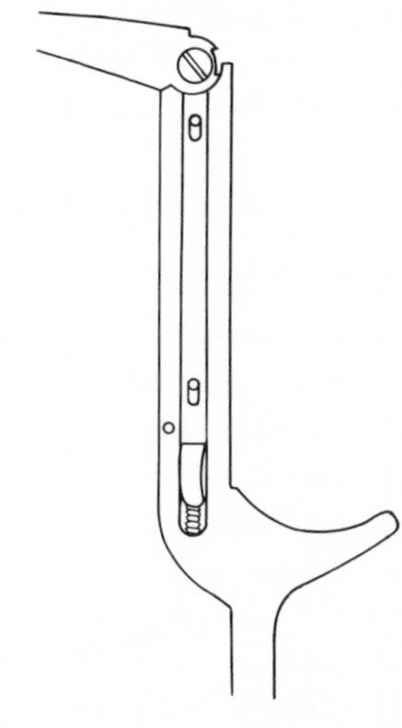

Fig. 5-5. Selective lock of Kielland-Barton forceps, disengaged.

When the lock is disengaged, the blade has mobility. Once the blade is returned to a position of alignment with the shank, the lock spontaneously snaps into place and the branch again is rigid. A small button on the surface of the shank near the handle prevents the sliding lock of the instrument from disengaging the spring lock.

Function

The primary function of the K-B forceps is rotation. Its secondary function is traction. The instrument is for the management of occiput transverse and posterior positions of the fetal head.

INSTRUMENTS FOR INCREASED TRACTION

The principle of axis-traction is a well-accepted component of all forceps deliveries. Although the clinician attempts to include this principle in his routine forceps extractions, there are instances which require the use of instrumental adjuncts to augment traction. Hence, it is imperative that he be familiar with axis-traction handles and at least one good axis-traction forceps.

The fifty years which followed Tarnier's monumental contribution of the axis-traction principle[101] produced an avalanche of forceps devoted to this concept. There were instruments whose traction handles had fixed or detachable wires, others with cloth or leather thongs. Some inventors preferred designing the axis-traction principle into accentuated curves within the shanks, while others added traction devices to already accepted instruments such as the Simpson and Elliott. A few, including DeWees and Dewey, concentrated on designing forceps exclusively for axis-traction. Although there are many acceptable axis-traction forceps, the Dewey is still a popular and efficient instrument when one needs a forceps to augment traction.

The Dewey Forceps

The axis-traction forceps introduced by Dewey at the turn of the century is a heavy, well-constructed instrument designed solely for the purpose of applying increased axis-traction. The instrument has an overall length of 37.5 cm. The blades are 17 cm. long, fenestrated, and slightly less tapered and thicker than those of the Simpson forceps in contour. The parallel shanks are 7 cm. in length and are separated 2 cm. (Fig. 5-6).

The locking mechanism of the Dewey forceps is of the German variety. Arising from the left shank is a fixed pin about which the right branch articulates. Behind this is a wing nut and screw which hinges across the shanks.

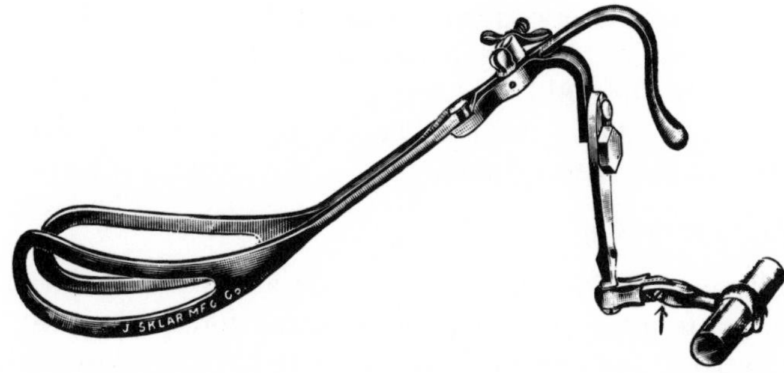

Fig. 5-6. Dewey forceps. *(Courtesy of J. Sklar Manufacturing Company.)*

The termination of each branch has been individualized. There are no traditional finger grips or handles. The right branch simply terminates in a downward curve. The left branch sharply angulates into a vertical portion which extends 4 cm. beneath the instrument. Attached to this by a large screw and elevated pin is the detachable vertical rod leading to the traction bar. The vertical bar has an overall length of 11 cm. but its line of traction occurs at 10 cm. beneath the bent handles. The horizontal traction bar is quite short, only 6 cm. in length. It articulates both with the vertical member and a transverse handle by rotary joints which are at right angles to each other. Midway on the traction bar is a simple hinge so that the transverse handle can be raised or lowered to the proper plane of traction. This plane is determined by lining up an arrowhead marker on the traction bar with a groove etched into either side of the hinge. The traction apparatus of the Dewey forceps is completely detachable.

Function

The Dewey forceps is a tractor. Although it may seem somewhat cumbersome to the novice and is difficult to apply because of its separated shanks, German lock, and unconventional handles, once the operator is familiar with it he develops great respect for the instrument. It is an excellent forceps when increased traction is needed for a large or well-molded head.

AXIS-TRACTION HANDLES

Most of the early traction forceps were greatly complicated by their wires and handles. It was for Stephenson of the University of Aberdeen in 1886 to find a simpler means of axis-traction which would be adaptable to any instrument. This he did by employing a simple hook which attached between the shanks and over the lock. The concept of a universal detachable traction handle reached ultimate fruition in 1924 when Bill[9] of Cleveland introduced his modification. The Bill handle allows the clinician to add accurate instrumental axis-traction to almost any forceps.

Bill Axis-Traction Handle

The Bill axis-traction handle consists of a claw which hooks over the finger grips and lock of any conventional forceps (*see* Fig. 2-15). A 7.5-cm. vertical rod extends from its lower surface. At its lower end the vertical rod articulates with the horizontal traction rod, which is 9 cm. in length. Where the vertical and traction rods join, there are lateral indicators resembling the point of an arrow. These are directed towards the traction rod and indicate the line of pull in which proper traction should be made. The traction rod terminates in a movable rotary joint which connects it to a cylindrical transverse handle. The apparatus can easily be removed either following delivery of the head or between pulls. The vertical and traction arms are of proper length so that a line drawn through the axis of the forceps' blades will be in direct continuity with the line of traction.

The instrument was designed to allow the clinician to employ traction in the proper plane of the pelvis. The movable joint where the vertical and traction rods meet allows the handles of the forceps to rise as traction is made and the head descends in the pelvis.

AFTERCOMING HEAD FORCEPS

The obstetrician's increasing awareness of the importance of proper management of breech presentation has stimulated interest in the control of the aftercoming head. Most students of the problem emphasize the use of prophylactic forceps here just as in vertex presentations. Despite the hundreds of forceps which have been invented, until recently only one instrument—the Piper forceps—had been designed specifically for this problem. Although some still prefer to use a more conventional instrument for the aftercoming head, the Piper has become the classic instrument for this complication. The longest of the modern obstetric forceps, it has recently been abbreviated and modified by the author.[56]

The Piper Forceps

In 1924 Edmund Piper of Philadelphia introduced his forceps for the management of the aftercoming head (*see* Fig. 1-10). The advantage of this instrument is a function of the long shanks which have a perineal curve. This allows for the handles to be at a lower level than the blades, making the forceps relatively easy to apply to the after-coming head from below.

Construction

Because of the light construction throughout its overall length of 44.5 cm., the instrument has a springlike quality. The hollow handles are 12 cm. in length and terminate in an English lock. The shanks, which rapidly diverge, are cylindrical, parallel, 3.5 cm. apart, and 15 cm. long. Throughout their length they have a gradual perineal curve. The fenestrated blades are 17.5 cm. long, 5 cm. in breadth, and have a very shallow cephalic curve. The slight pelvic curve of the blades becomes functional when the forceps is applied. Because of the length of the lever arm beyond the fulcrum, the separated shanks, and the shallow blades, compression of the fetal head is reduced with the Piper forceps.

The Short Piper Forceps

In 1967 after a ten-year clinical trial, the author introduced his modification of the Piper forceps.[56] The object was to create a true outlet forceps for the aftercoming head.

Construction

The essential modifications of the short Piper forceps are: shortening of the shanks to 11 cm.; replacement of the handles with transverse finger grips; and the insertion of a pivot articulation for the English lock (Fig. 5-7). The pivot lock eliminates crossing of the branches and

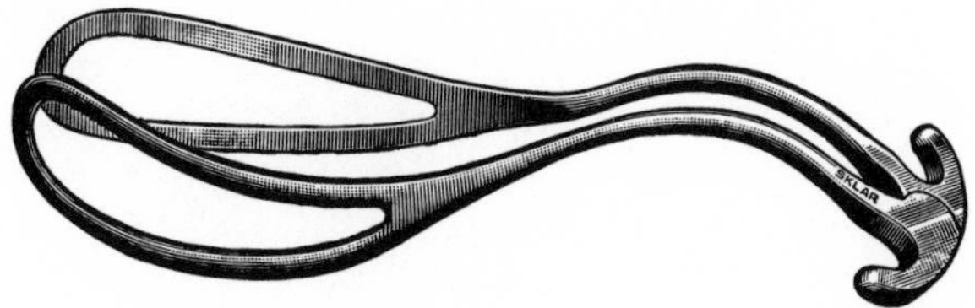

Fig. 5-7. Short Piper forceps. *(Courtesy of J. Sklar Manufacturing Company.)*

allows for a simple pelvic application of the forceps from beneath the fetal body. Since the pivot joint has mobility, the blades will fit any sized head. The pivot lock and finger grips convert the instrument into a third-class lever and eliminate compression of the fetal head unless the shanks are squeezed. All lateral compressive force will be derived from the maternal tissues. Because of its reduced overall length of 30 cm., the instrument is easy to maneuver compared to the classic Piper forceps, which tends to be unwieldy. Another advantage of the short Piper forceps is that the fetal body will rest gently on the shanks and over the operator's hand and wrists, affording better control.

Function

Both the classic and short Piper forceps are tractors. Traction with these instruments is augmented by elevation of the handles or finger grips. This produces flexion of the fetal head with subsequent delivery.

There are numerous other excellent special instruments for traction and rotation. Many have achieved popularity on a regional basis, i.e., the Boston or Chicago school. This selectivity stems from the tendency of senior clinicians to emphasize a special instrument with which they themselves had been indoctrinated. The above-mentioned forceps, however, will provide the obstetrician with more than ample instrumentation to deal with the complicated vaginal delivery.

Chapter Six

The Use of Obstetric Forceps

The obstetric forceps is a surgical instrument. Peculiar to our specialty, it is also unique in that it simultaneously relates to two patients. The clinician must be knowledgeable not only regarding the instrument's construction, function, and limitations, but he must be equally familiar with the indications and prerequisites for its use. If not, he can inflict rather than avoid damage to either or both of his patients.

As with any other surgical procedure, a forceps operation must be conducted in a proper setting. A delivery suite should not be one with fewer facilities than an operating area. In fact it should be a fully equipped operating area with the addition of special instrumentation. Every facility for major anesthesia and surgery must be available. The obstetrician should be able to perform an emergency section without having to move the patient or wait for the instruments to come from another area. Supportive adjuncts such as parenteral fluids should be within easy reach. Special instruments such as those needed for inspection of the genital tract must be in each delivery room. Each room must also contain appropriate facilities and means to care for, support, and resuscitate the newborn. In short, valuable time must not be lost to mother or child while personnel scurry about seeking equipment which is needed immediately.

When properly equipped and staffed, a delivery room will offer reassurance to both patient and physician that any eventuality can be handled. In such an environment, an obstetric delivery will achieve the dignity and safety it deserves.

INDICATIONS FOR OBSTETRIC FORCEPS

There are two kinds of indications for the use of obstetric forceps: maternal and fetal. The maternal indications are those systemic diseases which limit her physical reserve, and frank or impending exhaustion. The latter may include insufficiency of the powers. In both instances, shortening of the second stage of labor is desirable. The fetal indications for the use of forceps are: fetal distress, arrests of rotation, certain abnormal positions, the aftercoming head, and selected cases of relative cephalopelvic disproportion.

Most forceps deliveries performed today can be categorized as "prophylactic." This concept, proposed by DeLee[22a] in 1920, struck the obstetric world with considerable effect. DeLee advocated prophylactic interference for both mother and child. The fetal head was to be spared prolonged pounding against the perineum. The mother was to be spared not only the physical exhaustion of the second stage, but unnecessary overstretching of her pelvic floor and adjacent tissues.

When fetal distress occurs, is detected, and vaginal delivery can be safely expedited, there is a real indication for the use of forceps.

Rotary arrests include occiput posterior and transverse arrests which fail to make progress after a reasonable period of observation. In most of these instances, the head is deflexed. This attitude must be corrected prior to rotation if an atraumatic delivery is to be accomplished.

Abnormal presentations amenable to forceps delivery include selected cases of face and brow presentations.

The practice of using forceps for the aftercoming head is one which has received increased attention. The availability of special instruments for this problem has extended the concept of prophylactic forceps.

Intervention with forceps for a relative cephalopelvic disproportion is the most difficult condition to assess. If it is due to certain rotary arrests or abnormal presentations which when corrected reduce the disproportion, there is no controversy regarding forceps use. Increased maternal soft-tissue resistance which is relieved by an extended episiotomy also produces no consternation. Maximal clinical acumen is necessary, however, when labor has been difficult, the pelvic capacity borderline, and the head extensively molded. Such borderline cases should be rare because of the safety of cesarean section. Nevertheless, if confronted with such a problem, one must utilize every diagnostic and supportive aid available. These include pelvimetry, fluid replacement, expectant observation, and appropriate analgesia and anesthesia. The value of another opinion cannot be minimized.

Such a dilemma can present the clinician with the problem of "trial forceps." Although such cases are extremely rare, the astute attendant may attempt the luxury of a trial vaginal delivery comfortable in the knowledge that cesarean section can still safely be performed. If he does not have control of the force he will apply with the forceps, then cesarean section is the immediate procedure of choice. But if he can utilize the forceps judiciously—mimicking and augmenting the forces of labor—vaginal delivery usually can be safely accomplished.

The term "trial forceps" implies a questionable outcome—successful or unsuccessful. The former is the completion of a vaginal delivery without undue injury to either mother or child. The latter implies that after the attempted use of forceps, they have been abandoned, since vaginal delivery could not be accomplished without injury. When trauma from obstetric forceps is inflicted to either mother or child, however, we have "failed forceps." In this instance, undue force has been applied with deleterious results, whether or not vaginal delivery has been accomplished.

PREREQUISITES FOR THE USE OF FORCEPS

Forceps operations, just as any other surgical procedure, must meet numerous criteria before they can be successfully accomplished. Although these criteria are interrelated, they can be categorized into three groups relating to the fetus, the mother, and the attendant. All of these factors, however, revert to the operator, who is solely responsible. He must ascertain fetal status, make certain that the prerequisites for protecting the maternal tissues have been fulfilled, and not extend himself beyond his knowledge of forceps and proper technic. If these preoperative forceps criteria are systematically checked, the operation will have a successful outcome.

Fetal Factors

The factors which relate to the fetus are its size, position, attitude, station, and the degree of molding. Accurate knowledge of the position and attitude of the head is mandatory in order to select the appropriate instrument and to achieve proper application. The head must be well engaged. If its position cannot be determined by palpation of the sutures and fontanelles, then one should palpate an ear. If this also proves unsatisfactory, then one should seek the supraorbital ridge. Well-molded and large heads dictate the use of forceps with long tapered blades, while average and minimally molded heads are better fit by blades having an increased cephalic curve. The station at which the forceps is to be applied can influence the choice of an instrument which accentuates axis-traction.

Maternal Factors

The maternal factors which are related to the successful accomplishment of a forceps delivery are the size, configuration, and capacity of the bony pelvis. These factors must be ascertained prior to the application of the forceps. An accurate knowledge of the pelvic capacity will indicate to the operator which of the pelvic diameters is most favorable for the safest and easiest completion of the delivery.

There are numerous soft-tissue factors which are also involved. The tension and thickness of the perineum must be evaluated so that the episiotomy can be performed at the opportune time before overstretching of the soft tissues occurs. The membranes must be ruptured. The bladder and rectum should not be full. The concept of routine catheterization prior to forceps delivery has been gradually abandoned in order to avoid the introduction of infection or bacteruria. When these hollow visci are distended, however, considerable trauma can be avoided to them if they are emptied prior to delivery, particularly when a midforceps rotation is anticipated. Not only must the cervix be completely dilated, it should be retracted over the fetal head. There are rare instances, such as midpelvic transverse arrest, where the operator can palpate an anterior lip of cervix. This is usually negotiable, however, and either can be gently pushed over the head or elevated in order that the forceps can be properly applied.

A most important consideration for the mother is the administration of an adequate anesthetic. Whether general, regional, or local it must be sufficient to allow the forceps to be applied and traction instituted without inducing discomfort and resistance.

Attendant Factors

The factors related to the attendant are: the ability to decide what the primary need of a given patient is, thorough knowledge of the forceps he selects, and the technical ability to properly use the instrument. Deciding what the primary need is—traction or rotation—will influence the choice of instrument. Unless capable of properly applying and employing a particular forceps, however, it is foolhardy to attempt to use it. In other words, the attendant must be able to properly use the instrument of his choice both within its limitations and his own.

CLASSIFICATION OF FORCEPS OPERATIONS

There are numerous classifications which describe forceps deliveries. These may vary not only from one area to another, but from one institution to another. Despite individual preferences, it seems logical that a uniform classification should be adopted. Only with such conformity can comparable data be developed. Perhaps the present classification of forceps deliveries will be altered by the evolution of new data from those individuals working with metric forceps and other recording devices. Until that time, however, it seems proper to accept the classification proposed in the *Manual of Standards* published by the American College of Obstetricians and Gynecologists.[63]

1. Outlet forceps: The application of forceps when the scalp is or has been visible at the introitus without separating the labia, the skull has reached the pelvic floor, and the sagittal suture is in the anteroposterior diameter of the pelvis.
2. Midforceps: The application of forceps when the head is engaged, but the conditions for outlet forceps have not been met. In the context of this term, any forceps delivery requiring artificial rotation regardless of the station from which extraction is begun, shall be designated a "midforceps" delivery. The term "low midforceps" is disapproved. A record shall be made of the position and the station of the head when the delivery is begun. In addition, a description of the various maneuvers, and of any difficulties encountered in the application of the forceps and in the extraction of the infant shall be recorded.
3. High forceps: The application of forceps at any time prior to full engagement of the head. High forceps delivery is almost never justifiable.

Review of this classification reveals that the terms "low forceps" and "low midforceps" have been deleted. The latter has become extremely popular with the advent and increasing use of conduction anesthesia, which so often leads to incomplete rotations of the fetal head. When it is used, the low midforceps category becomes an inviting catchall for true midforceps rotations and extractions. As stated, the term "outlet forceps" means the true outlet extraction of a direct occiput anterior or posterior. When there is need for rotation prior to extraction, the vertex has not reached the pelvic floor and a "midforceps" operation has been performed.

Midforceps operations should be adequately described by the position and station of the head as well as any maneuver involved. Special notation is encouraged for any difficulties encountered. Many authorities have urged describing the difficulty of traction as minimal, moderate, or maximal.

It has been estimated that more than one-third of the deliveries in this country are accomplished with the assistance of obstetric forceps. The past decade has witnessed an avid interest in the long-range outcome of this multitude of operative procedures on the newborn. If meaningful results are to be derived from this data, not only accurate but complete records must be kept. In order to facilitate the recording of the pertinent data of a forceps delivery, a relatively simple delivery record can be utilized (Fig. 6-1). This information should augment the standard information recorded regarding labor and delivery.

This form includes space for recording the category of forceps delivery, instrument and anesthetic used, position and station of the fetal head, special maneuvers employed, degrees of rotation, and an evaluation of the amount of traction required.

FORCEPS DELIVERY RECORD

	Outlet	Mid	High
Position			
Station			
Rotation			

Traction Minimal ☐ Moderate ☐ Maximum ☐

Forceps ____________ Anesthetic ____________ Maneuver ____________

Signature ____________________

Fig. 6-1. Forceps delivery record.

The data to be recorded is easily standardized. The traditional nomenclature which describes position, station, and degrees of rotation should be used. Traction should be described as minimal, moderate, or maximal. For instance, an ROA rotated 45° to an OA and delivered with minimal traction with Tucker-McLane forceps from a +3 station would indicate an easy forceps delivery. On the other hand, an LOT rotated 90° and delivered with Kielland forceps and moderate traction from 0 station is indicative of a much more difficult procedure. Under maneuver, the attendant records such things as the Scanzoni procedure or type of application when such instruments as the Kielland forceps are used. The extra minute or so required of the obstetrician to complete such a record may have significant meaning in the future evaluation of forceps procedures.

*

Chapter Seven

*

Outlet Forceps Technics

*

By definition, outlet forceps are those applied to the fetal head which has reached the pelvic floor, whose scalp is or has been visible at the introitus, and whose sagittal suture is in the anteroposterior diameter of the pelvis. Outlet forceps procedures constitute the great majority of forceps operations and can be categorized as prophylactic. As such, they are for traction only. Once rotation is included, the operation can no longer be classified as an outlet one.

The outlet forceps operation is the simplest of forceps operations, but it still demands complete adherence to all of the prerequisites. As with any other operative procedure, it must be conducted in a proper sequential manner. The factors involved are choice of appropriate instrument, application and articulation of the branches, traction, and removal of the forceps.

CHOICE OF INSTRUMENT

Once the operator has decided that the use of outlet forceps is indicated and that the prerequisites for their use are satisfied, he must select an appropriate instrument. The conventional forceps fall into two major categories, depending upon the contour of the blades. The Simpson forceps and its modifications with their long, shallow, tapered blades are most suitable to large and extensively molded fetal heads. The Elliott forceps and its modifications with their shorter blades and accentuated cephalic curve are more suitable to the rounded fetal head which has not undergone extensive molding.

Other factors also influence the choice of instrument. Many prefer the Elliott-type instruments because of their overlapping shanks, which do not distend the perineum as do the separated shanks of the Simpson-type forceps. A most popular instrument is the Tucker-McLane with Luikart modification. This instrument offers the advantages of overlapping shanks and the Elliott blade contour with pseudofenestration for easy application and firm grasp of the fetal head. When a short blade with increased cephalic curve is desired, the author prefers his divergent forceps since it minimizes compression and enhances traction with the perineal curve in its shanks.

One must remember that there is no perfect instrument. Each type has inherent advantages and disadvantages and an appropriate place in outlet deliveries. When the blades fit the head well, no pressure points will be created nor will there be slippage. If by chance the operator has selected a forceps which does not fit the fetal head well, it is better to change instruments prior to traction. Otherwise there is an increased possibility of inflicting trauma to mother and child.

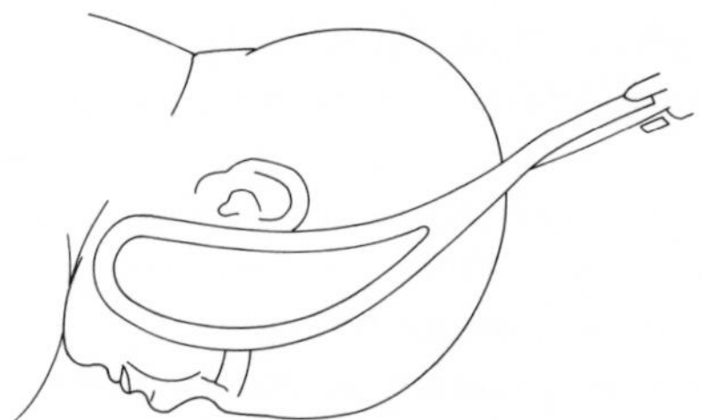

Fig. 7-1. Cephalic (bimalar-biparietal) forceps application.

No matter which forceps has been selected for use, application and articulation of the branches must be made properly. For this to be accomplished, accurate identification of the landmarks of the fetal skull is mandatory. The sagittal suture and both fontanelles must be identified. Errors are invited by a hasty diagnosis of position on the basis of a single landmark. Once certain of the position, the operator must constantly keep in mind that he wants to achieve an accurate *cephalic* application of the blades. This is defined as a bimalar-biparietal application of the blades which will evenly distribute the force to be applied (Fig. 7-1). Accuracy of the application must be confirmed prior to traction. There should be no pressure points.

A *pelvic* application of the forceps is acceptable only for the aftercoming head, since there is no opportunity to identify the usual landmarks.

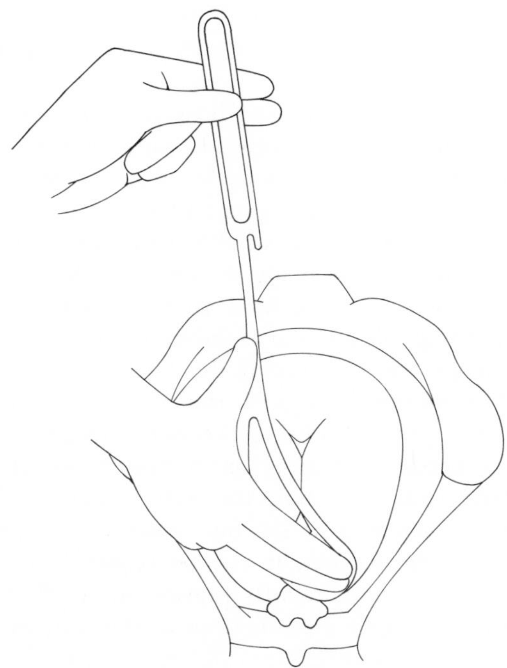

Fig. 7-2. Occiput anterior, insertion of the left branch.

OCCIPUT ANTERIOR

The first step in the application of obstetric forceps is the insertion of the branches into the vagina. It is always wise to orient the forceps to the position they will occupy in the pelvis once applied. Presuming that a classic forceps is being used for an occiput anterior position, the left branch should be inserted first. This will facilitate articulation since the lock is usually on the left branch. If the right branch were inserted first, the shanks and handles would have to be recrossed to achieve proper articulation.

The insertion of the left branch is begun by creating a space between the fetal head and the pelvic wall. The prelubricated middle and index fingers of the right hand are inserted into the vagina along the left side of the fetal head. This not only reconfirms that the cervix is fully retracted, but provides a shield for the maternal soft tissues.

The left branch, with its blade prelubricated, is now oriented for insertion. The handle is held upright, slightly toward the right maternal groin, as if it were a pen or pencil (Fig. 7-2). This makes the shank almost perpendicular to the floor and orients the pelvic and cephalic curves of the blades to their intended course. The right thumb is now placed at the heel of the blade. By allowing the shank to slide over the thumb, the downward descent of the branch is controlled.

The handle is now gently lowered in a sweeping arc which begins toward the operator's left and ends at the midline when the shank and handle reach a horizontal position. No force should be applied at the handle; the branch should descend almost completely by the force of gravity. The rate of descent of the shank and handle, and thus the force of insertion of the blade, is controlled by the right thumb. During this maneuver, the blade is guided upward into the pelvis along its pelvic curve. In response to the arc of the handle, the cephalic curve of the blade courses around the fetal head toward a proper cephalic application. Once applied, the branch usually will be held in place by pelvic pressure so that the right branch can be inserted. When there is pelvic relaxation, as in multiparas, it is sometimes necessary to have an assistant hold the branch in place.

If the operator feels that he has not achieved a proper application of this branch of the forceps, it can be adjusted without removal. Prominent ischial spines frequently prevent the blade from attaining a bimalar-biparietal application in front of the fetal ear. Adjustment

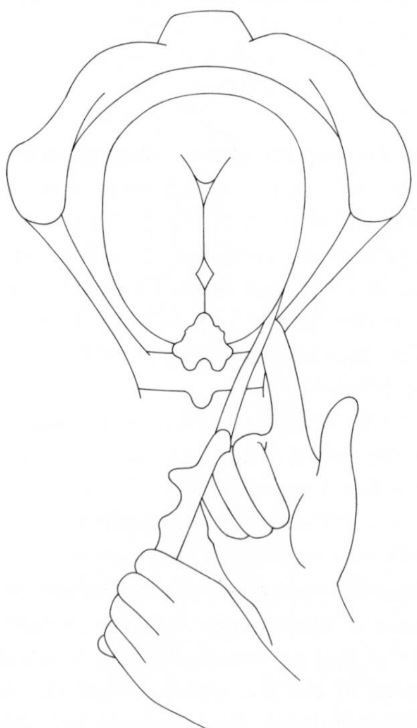

Fig. 7-3. Occiput anterior, adjustment of the left branch.

is performed with the handle held in the left hand and the right index finger beneath the shank at the heel of the blade (Fig. 7-3). The handle is slightly depressed as the finger elevates and orients the blade to the desired application. Once again, most of the force is derived from the finger beneath the blade rather than from the hand on the handle.

Once the left branch has been inserted into the vagina and applied to the fetal head, the right branch is applied. This is accomplished in an identical manner as the left, but with the hands and maneuvers reversed. Adjustment of this branch may also be necessary and is accomplished the same way.

The next step following the introduction and application of the branches is their articulation. It is most tempting for the inexperienced operator to use this step as a means of adjusting blade application. This must never be done if trauma is to be avoided. Proper application must be achieved prior to articulation. The locking of the branches should be accomplished in an almost effortless manner. If resistance to locking of the branches is encountered, their application and relationship must be rechecked and adjusted. Easy locking is frequently facilitated by equal depression of the handles.

Once the branches are locked, it is important not to squeeze the handles, or increased compression will result. There is no need for the handles to be in close approximation to accomplish delivery.

Now the operator must accurately ascertain the application of the forceps he has achieved. The standards for this are:

1. The sagittal suture must be equidistant between the branches. If the shanks are parallel, the sagittal suture should be midway between them; if overlapping, directly in line with them.
2. The posterior fontanelle should be one finger's breadth above the shanks.
3. If the blades are fenestrated, they should admit one finger between the heel of the blade and the fetal head.

TRACTION

Traction is the only function of outlet forceps. It must not be initiated, however, until the forceps has been properly applied and its relationship with the fetal head confirmed. Traction is best accomplished with the operator in a sitting position. He should be at a comfortable level so that his flexed forearms are slightly beneath the level of the delivery table. The forceps should be grasped from beneath and all traction generated should be derived from the forearm. If additional force is applied, the operator has engaged the infant and mother in a contest of strength—with the losers predictable.

Nothing should obstruct the operator's vision of the field. He must constantly observe the descent and extension of the head as well as the distention of the perineum in order to perform an episiotomy at the most opportune time. If indicated, this is usually done prior to maximal stretching of the perineum in order to spare overstretching and tearing of the deeper tissues. At this time, there is less chance to injure the rectum, and blood loss is minimized thanks to compression of the vessels.

As with every other forceps procedure, traction must be performed in a prescribed manner. It must follow the curve of the pelvis, and it must be accomplished in a sequence of controlled efforts.

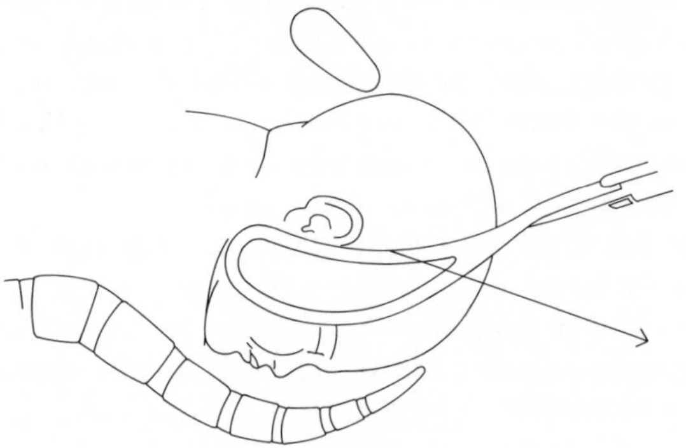

Fig. 7-4. Traction in the axis of the pelvis, outlet forceps.

All traction must be carried out in a plane continuous with the curve of the pelvis. This implies a downward pull, the angle of which increases the higher the station of the head. Although the angle is slight with outlet forceps, traction still must be performed in the proper axis (Fig. 7-4). With conventional forceps that have straight shanks, traction in the plane of the pelvic curve is achieved by the Saxtorph-Pajot maneuver.

In 1771 Saxtorph recognized that much of the force of horizontal traction was expended against the symphysis. To achieve an axis of pull continuous with the pelvic curve, he advocated a bimanual procedure. Downward vertical pressure is applied to the shanks with one hand, while the other hand applies a straight pull on the handles. Properly performed, this maneuver results in a vector continuous with the central pelvic axis. Later popularized by Pajot, it has become known as the Saxtorph-Pajot maneuver.

Excellent control of this maneuver can be developed by placing the index and middle fingers of the left hand over the shanks while the handles are grasped from beneath by the right hand (Fig. 7-5). If the instrument has parallel separated shanks, the third finger can be inserted between them to act as a cushion. The adjacent fingers rest over the finger grips of the handles and compression is reduced. If the instrument has overlapping shanks, it is the index and middle fingers which hook over the finger grips of the handles.

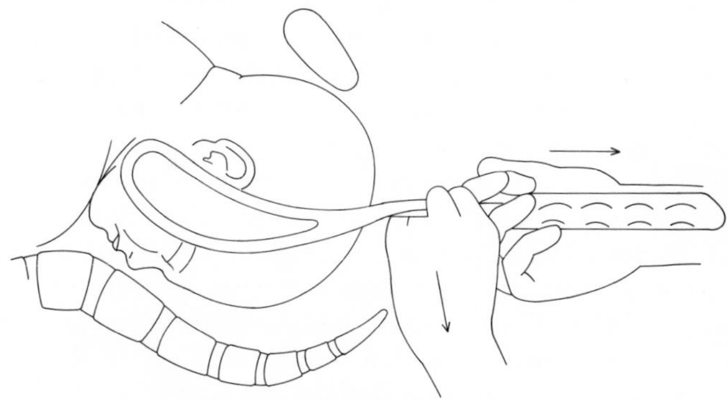

Fig. 7-5. Saxtorph-Pajot maneuver.

The performance of a forceps extraction consists of a series of tractive efforts. Each pull should begin gradually, reach an acme of intensity, be sustained for a short but definite interval, and then gradually subside. Traction should mimic and augment the force of labor. Jerking must be avoided. There must be a definite interval of rest between pulls, at which time the forceps should be unlocked to eliminate continuous compression.

The first tractive effort is known as the *trial traction*. It should indicate to the operator how much resistance exists and how much effort will have to be expended. It also provides an opportunity to recheck the accuracy of the forceps application. If there is concern regarding fetal status, the interval following the trial traction should be used to check the fetal heart tones.

As the series of tractive efforts is initiated, the fingers depressing the shanks act as a guide to the path of least resistance. If the occiput seems to be impeded by the symphysis, increased force on the shanks is required. If the pelvic floor seems to be presenting resistance, the force on the shanks should be reduced. One must remember that there is no predetermined number of tractive pulls nor is there a time limitation in a normal delivery.

Once the operator observes the occiput pass beneath the pubic angle, he alters the course of the forceps. Since the head delivers by extension, it is this mechanism which must now be augmented. This is accomplished by the gradual steady elevation of the handles to an angle of about 40° above the horizontal. By this action, the head is lifted over the perineum. The maneuver can be performed either by lifting the forceps with a single finger at the crotch of the shanks, or by continuous elevation of the finger grips.

Once the biparietal diameter of the head has passed the vulvar ring, the forceps can be removed. The operator may desire to control the head by a modified Ritgen maneuver to prevent recession. In most primiparas, however, recession of the head rarely occurs once the biparietal diameter of the head has delivered. The forceps is unlocked and the branches removed in reverse order of their application. Each branch must again pass through a sweeping curve toward the opposite maternal groin so that the cephalic curve of the blade will course around the fetal head. Although infrequent, difficulty in removal of the forceps is most often encountered with instruments that have fenestrated blades. The forceps should never be removed by force. If resistance is met, removal of each branch may be aided by applying lateral pressure to the inner surface of the heel of the blade. If this does not assist in their easy removal, one or both branches should be allowed to remain properly applied and then removed following completion of the delivery of the head.

Some of the newer forceps, because of their special design, warrant consideration for outlet forceps deliveries. The Hawks-Dennen forceps, with its built-in axis-traction principle in the shanks, eliminates the need for the Saxtorph-Pajot maneuver.[26,27] It provides the operator with the proper inclination of traction by its angulated shanks.

With parallel or divergent forceps, one must remember that the branches do not cross. The blade which fits the right side of the head will have its handle or finger grip in the operator's left hand.

The author's divergent forceps is inserted in the usual manner, but because of its reduced length does not require an extensive sweeping curve of the shanks. After both branches are applied, the pivot lock is engaged. Articulation frequently requires depression of the finger grips to carefully align the shanks, since the slot for the pivot lock is narrow. This has an advantage, however, because the absence of vertical mobility in the lock assures a symmetrical application of the blades. The axle of the lock allows the branches to pivot easily, which assures a proper fit for any sized head. Proper plane of pull is obtained by traction in a line continuous with the perineal curve of the shanks. As traction is instituted and the head passes beneath the pubic angle,

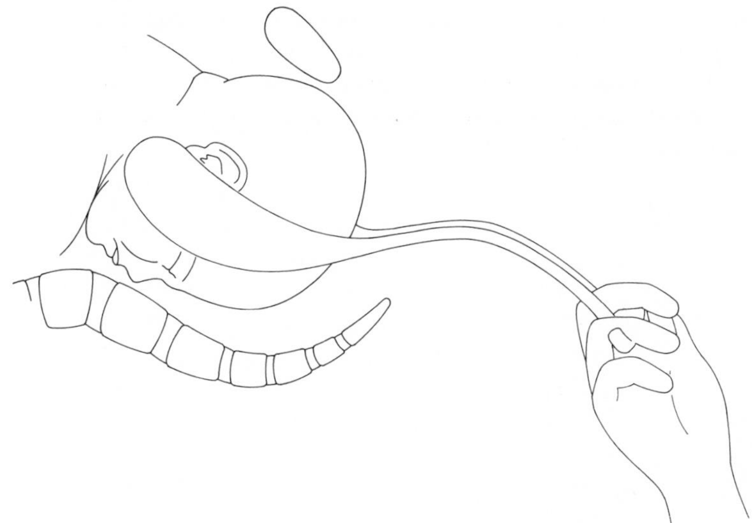

Fig. 7-6. Application and traction, divergent forceps.

the shanks diverge so that the blades derive their compression from the pelvic walls.

Extension of the head with this forceps is accomplished by merely elevating the finger grips in an arc to about 30° above the horizontal (Fig. 7-6). Because of its divergent ability and lack of compression, removal can be deferred until the head has been delivered. Experience with the instrument proves this to be the easiest course.

OCCIPUT POSTERIOR

When forceps are used to deliver an occiput posterior which meets the criteria for outlet forceps, certain relationships change. Although the technic for insertion and application of the branches is essentially identical to that used for an occiput anterior, the blades fit the opposite side of the fetal head. The left branch, which fits the left side of the pelvis, is now in apposition to the right side of the fetal head and the right branch, the left side of the head. One must remember that the widest diameter (biparietal) of the fetal head is in the posterior segment of the pelvis. Hence, increased care must be taken to bring the blades around the parietal bosses and achieve proper application.

With an occiput posterior, the pelvic curve of the blades is reversed in its relationship to the fetal head. When applied to an occiput anterior, the toes of the blades curve toward the ears. Applied to an occiput posterior, the toes of the blades curve away from the ears and toward the mouth. For this reason it is wise to use a forceps with tapered Simpson-type blades to avoid pressure points on the soft tissues of the face. The Hawks-Dennen forceps is particularly suitable for this type of delivery (Fig. 7-7).

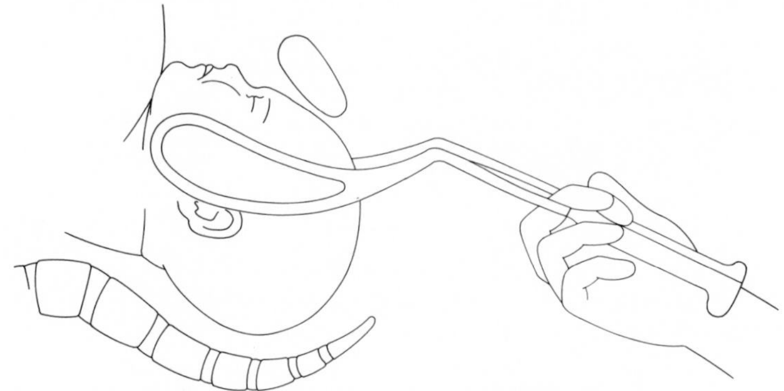

Fig. 7-7. Occiput posterior, Hawks-Dennen forceps application.

There is also a major change in the relationship of the forceps to the landmarks of the skull. The posterior fontanelle will be one finger's breadth beneath, rather than above, the shanks. This relationship must be confirmed prior to instituting traction to an occiput posterior.

Traction to an occiput posterior is performed as with an occiput anterior. One must remember, however, that since the largest part of the fetal head is in the posterior pelvic segment, increased distention of the perineum will occur. Therefore, a liberal episiotomy should be made a little earlier than usual. A median episiotomy is usually avoided, because extension into the rectum is more likely to occur with an occiput posterior.

The mechanism of delivery of the head is also reversed in occiput posteriors. Flexion, rather than extension, delivers the occiput over the perineum. Once this has occurred, the chin will deliver beneath the pubic symphysis. The blades are then removed in the usual manner and the delivery is completed.

Chapter Eight

Basic Midforceps

*

As a convenience, basic midforceps operations will be classified as those which require increased axis-traction or require less than a 90° rotation of the head. When a forceps rotation of 90° or greater is required, we are dealing with a major midforceps procedure, for which there are numerous special instruments and maneuvers. These are individually described in Chapters 9 and 10. Forceps rotations of 45° from either an LOA or ROA are quite frequent because of the increased use of conduction anesthesia.

LEFT OCCIPUT ANTERIOR (LOA)

A cardinal rule for the insertion and application of forceps to a vertex in an oblique pelvic diameter is that the posterior blade must be inserted first. For an LOA this is the left branch. The technic for insertion is basically identical to that described for a direct occiput anterior. The handle is held lightly in the left hand and the right creates the vaginal path which the blade is to follow. Insertion is begun by orienting the handle toward the right maternal groin, with the blade directed toward the left posterior segment of the pelvis. By guiding the blade along the course of the left posterior pelvis, it is directed around the curve of the fetal head and attains a position in front of the left ear (Fig. 8-1). Proper cephalic application of this branch can thus immediately be achieved. It is always imperative to allow the handle and shank to describe their descending arc without applying force through the left hand. The right thumb governs the force of insertion as the shank slides over it.

If a proper cephalic application has been achieved, the shank will be parallel to the left oblique diameter of the pelvis. The branch will

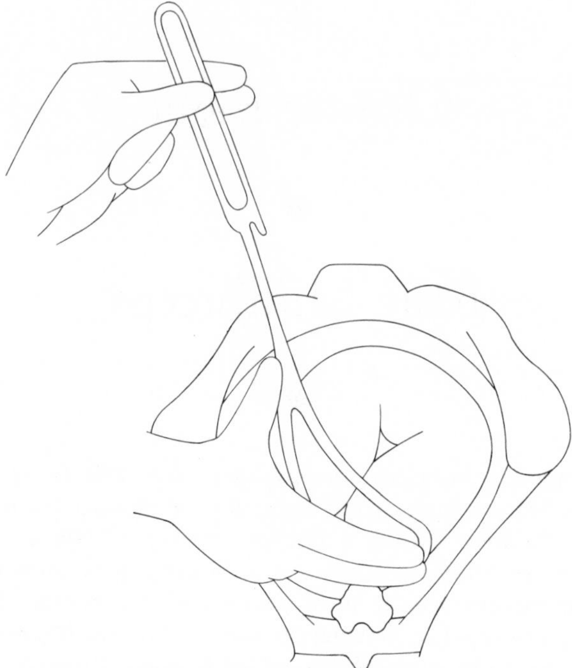

Fig. 8-1. Insertion of left (posterior) branch, LOA.

usually maintain its proper position because of the natural internal pelvic pressure. In multiparas, it is more likely that the branch will move and therefore it must be held in place by an assistant.

To insert the anterior or right branch, the hands are reversed; i.e., the right hand grasps the handle and the left hand is inserted into the vagina. Since the right blade must be directed toward the right anterior segment of the pelvis, the toe of the blade must be oriented in this direction. Consequently, the descending lateral arc of the handle and branch must be increased (Fig. 8-2). This will reduce the degree of wandering which must be done to achieve proper application of the blade. With proper application, the right shank also will be parallel to the left oblique diameter of the pelvis.

If resistance should be met, and the blade consequently inserted either to the posterior or lateral aspect of the right side of the pelvis, it must be adjusted by wandering it up and over the brow. This is accomplished with the left index and middle fingers elevating the shank, and the right hand depressing the handle downward and laterally. If the operator meets resistance to wandering the blade, he should

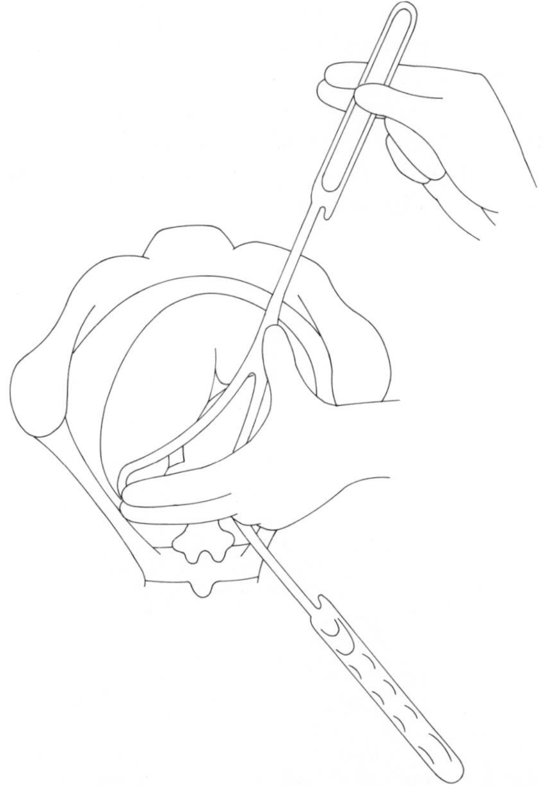

Fig. 8-2. Insertion of right (anterior) branch, LOA.

insert the left hand into the vagina before attempting to apply any increased force at the handle. He can thus protect the vaginal wall and help to guide the blade into its proper cephalic relationship.

Once both branches are properly applied, the branches are locked. It is not necessary to bring the handles into direct apposition, but only to achieve a secure articulation (Fig. 8-3).

Three cardinal points of the forceps application must now be checked. These must be verified prior to attempting rotation or applying traction. They are the adequacy of forceps insertion, the symmetry of application, and the accuracy of blade-cephalic relationship.

To verify the *adequacy of the forceps insertion,* the heels or fenestrations of the blades must be checked. The depth of insertion of a solid blade is evaluated by palpating the length of the heel which is in advance of the head. The length must be identical for both branches. With a fenestrated instrument, it is much easier to check the adequacy of insertion. The operator should be able to insert the tip of the index finger into the portion of the fenestration which is in advance of the head. If more than one finger can be inserted into the fenestration, the depth of insertion is inadequate. Inadequate insertion of the branches makes for an improper fit of the blades. If traction or rotation is then attempted, not only will pressure points be created on the soft tissues of the face, but the blades will tend to pull off.

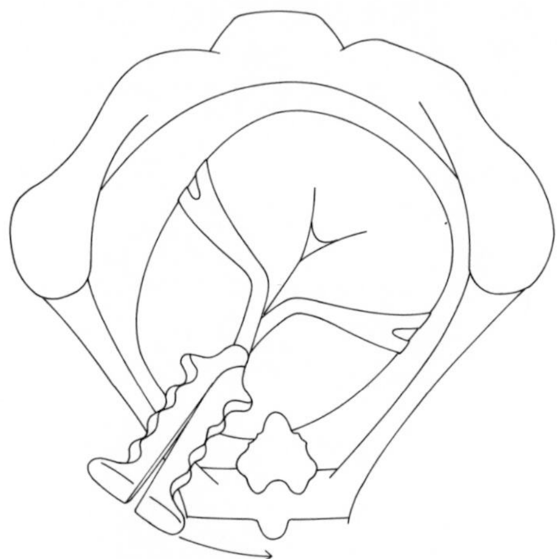

Fig. 8-3. Application and rotation of forceps, LOA.

To check the *symmetry of application,* the relationship of the sagittal suture to the shanks of the blades is evaluated. The suture must be midway between the blades. If the sagittal suture is not midway between the branches, the forceps have been applied in a brow-mastoid relationship. This must be corrected immediately to avoid the pressure points on the soft tissues of the face. The handles should be unlocked and the blades loosened. It is usually not necessary to remove the forceps, but one or both branches can be removed if the application is especially erratic and resistance is encountered in the adjustment. Most commonly it is the anterior or right blade which must be adjusted. This is accomplished by raising the shank with the middle or index finger of the left hand and depressing the handle with the right hand in order to elevate the blade and allow it to progress forward toward the anterior ear. Poor application of the left or posterior blade is usually due to a deep insertion. This is adjusted by a gradual withdrawal of the branch until the plane of its shank is at right angles with the sagittal suture. Once the blades have been readjusted, the handles are relocked and the relationship of the branches with the sagittal suture checked again.

The third cardinal check point is the *accuracy of blade-cephalic relationship.* This is determined by evaluating the position of the posterior fontanelle in relation to the shanks. It should be one finger's breadth above the shanks. If the posterior fontanelle is found to be more than one finger's breadth anterior to the plane of the shanks, the branches must be elevated. This can be accomplished only after they have been unlocked. They are then elevated one at a time to the proper level. If the posterior fontanelle has been found to be less than a finger's breadth above the plane of the shanks or even beneath the shanks, the unlocked handles should be depressed until the shanks reach the desired relationship with the posterior fontanelle. Once relocked, their relationship with the posterior fontanelle must be checked again.

The operator must remember that with any error of insertion or application, each or both branches can be completely removed and the forceps reapplied. This is a much safer course to follow when there is any doubt or when resistance is encountered in achieving a proper fit. By removing the branches, there will be better opportunity to completely reevaluate the status and position of the fetal head.

RIGHT OCCIPUT ANTERIOR (ROA)

The technic for the insertion, application, and articulation of the forceps for an ROA is similar to that for an LOA, except that the branches are reversed. The right branch becomes the posterior one and is the first to be inserted and applied. This is performed with the handle oriented toward the left maternal groin and controlled by the right hand. The left hand creates the space in the vagina for the insertion and application of the blade. Then the anterior or left branch is inserted and applied. Only one modification in the technic is necessary. Since the locking mechanism of conventional forceps is usually English style and on the left shank, the branches must be recrossed before they can be locked. The shanks are separated and the left handle is passed beneath the right to achieve articulation.

ROTATION AND EXTRACTION

To orient the fetal head to the anterior posterior diameter of the pelvis from an ROA or LOA, it must be rotated 45° toward the midline. This should require minimal force and be performed in a gradual manner, allowing the maternal tissues and fetal head to adapt to the new position. Rotation is performed by slightly elevating the handles through an arc in the desired direction. Once the anteroposterior plane of the pelvis has been reached, the cardinal landmarks are again checked to determine that slippage of the blades has not occurred.

Assured of his forceps application following rotation, the operator now proceeds with the extraction. Traction is applied with the Saxtorph-Pajot maneuver as described for outlet forceps. If the vertex should be at a higher pelvic station, increased depression of the shanks is necessary to augment traction in the true curve of the pelvis.

On rare occasions, it is desirable to deliver the baby in one of the oblique diameters of the pelvis. If the pelvis tends toward the android type or the coccyx is markedly prominent or anteflexed (anthropoid), an oblique diameter will afford an easier and less traumatic route for extraction. Even if the head has reached the anterior posterior diameter, it can be rotated 45° to an LOA or ROA in order to utilize a more desirable plane in such cases.

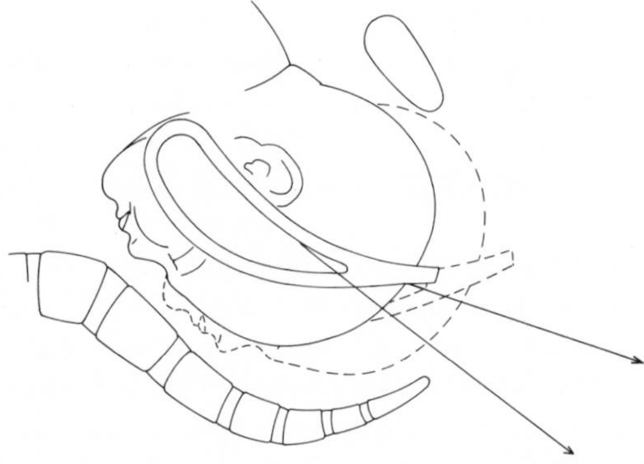

Fig. 8-4. Traction in the axis of the pelvis depending on station.

INSTRUMENTAL AXIS-TRACTION

Increased instrumental axis-traction can be a valuable adjunct in the management of large babies, late failure of the powers of labor, or midpelvic arrests due to conduction anesthesia. One must remember that the direction of axis-traction is related to the station at which it is instituted. The higher the station, the greater the angle of traction (Fig. 8-4).

With an average-sized infant and the vertex at midpelvis, axis-traction is best augmented by the addition of the Bill traction handle to the forceps of choice (Fig. 8-5). The attendant can apply traction in the proper plane by following the lateral markers. It is wise that this, too, be accomplished in a gradual manner. Between traction pulls, the Bill handle should be loosened or removed to allow the handles and blades to separate. This reduces prolonged compression of the fetal head. There is no need to implement axis-traction by additional pull via the shanks and handles of the forceps. As the occiput impinges beneath the symphysis, the traction handle is raised in a sweeping arc to accomplish extension of the head. Once this occurs, the handle should be removed and the delivery completed in routine fashion.

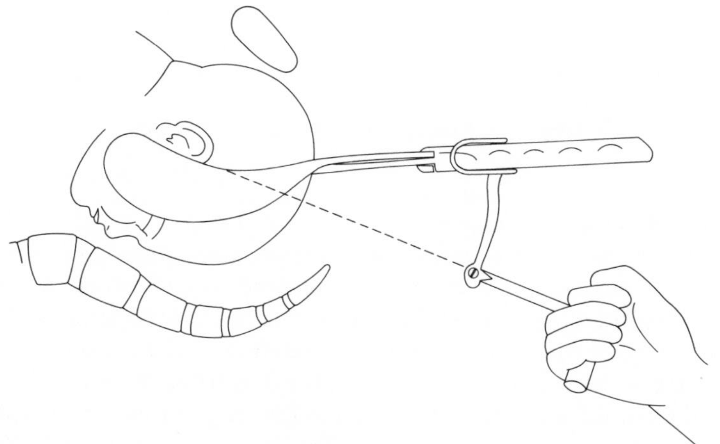

Fig. 8-5. Instrumental axis-traction, using Tucker-McLane forceps with Bill traction handle.

When one is dealing with a well-molded or a large head, an axis-traction instrument with long tapered blades (Simpson type) is most desirable. A forceps whose blades have an increased cephalic curve (Elliott type) will create pressure points at the toes of the blades, resulting in soft-tissue trauma to the face. The Dewey forceps fulfills the criteria for an instrument to manage these problems. Its tapered fenestrated blades assure a secure and proper fit to large or well-molded heads. Although heavy and perhaps a little cumbersome, if properly used, the Dewey will provide excellent instrumental axis-traction.

The Dewey forceps is inserted, applied, and adjusted in the usual manner. Limited rotation, if necessary, can also be performed. Care must be taken with the German lock. If the wing nut is excessively

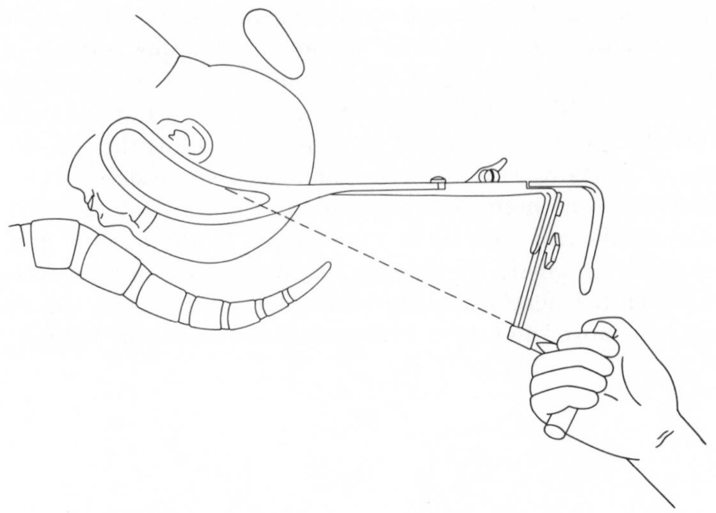

Fig. 8-6. Axis-traction with Dewey forceps.

tightened, increased compression will occur. It should be tightened only enough to achieve a secure application and shoud be released between traction pulls to avoid sustained compression. An early liberal episiotomy is advisable, since the separated parallel shanks produce early and marked perineal stretching. All traction with this instrument should be applied through the traction handle (Fig. 8-6).

Although infrequently indicated, the Dewey or a comparable forceps is an invaluable aid when increased axis-traction is required for the management of midpelvic arrests of large or well-molded heads.

*

Chapter Nine

*

Occiput Transverse Positions

*

Transverse position of the fetal head is one of the major complications which can be amenable to forceps delivery. This problem has consistently attracted the attention of obstetricians and has prompted innumerable reviews. It has also spurred many efforts to devise special maneuvers and forceps for its management. No procedure, however, can substitute for cesarean section when indicated. In order to manage this problem from below, each patient must be analyzed individually, since the etiology varies. The obstetrician must determine the cause of the arrest and decide what he wishes to accomplish—rotation and/or traction—and if both, in what sequence. He must then select an appropriate instrument to achieve his purpose.

True transverse arrests can be classified as "high" or "low." In the former, the arrest has occurred above the midpelvis and in almost all such instances, cesarean section is the procedure of choice. Low or deep transverse arrests are those in which the vertex has failed to progress beyond the +2 station following an adequate trial of second stage labor. Unless there is a true outlet contracture in these cases, vaginal delivery usually can be accomplished without trauma.

The problem of transverse arrest can occur in any type of pelvis. In a flat pelvis, it may be the normal mechanism of delivery. The prominent sacrum of an android type pelvis may inhibit internal rotation of a transverse head. In the gynecoid or anthropoid pelvis, late failure of the powers during the second stage of labor will prevent complete anterior rotation from the transverse or posterior position of engagement.

A frequent cause of transverse position in the multipara is the increased size of successive babies. A large infant in a normal pelvis can produce a borderline disproportion at the spines and result in late inertia and arrest. Another cause is the premature use of conduction anesthesia, which predisposes to incomplete rotation. Although the fetal head is not truly arrested, the attendant must face the problem of accomplishing a 90° rotation prior to extraction.

Both manual and instrumental procedures are available for the operative management of transverse positions and arrests. Instrumental procedures can be performed with either conventional forceps or the special forceps designed for the management of this problem. One must remember that a slight deflexion of the fetal head is inherent in transverse positions and must be corrected prior to any rotary maneuver.

MANUAL ROTATION

Manual rotation, like any other surgical procedure, should be accomplished in the simplest fashion possible. There are a series of increasingly complex maneuvers which the obstetrician may employ. Deflexion can be corrected by the Hodge maneuver—direct pressure to the sinciput, which will increase flexion. Occasionally, if uterine contractions are still present, this will result in spontaneous rotation.

The next maneuver which can be attempted is performed by the introduction of the middle and index fingers to the anterior frontal parietal area. For an LOT, the operator inserts the middle and index fingers of his left hand in front of the right ear and attempts rotation by simple downward pressure. The right hand acts as an external aid in pushing the right shoulder toward the midline. Once rotation occurs, the right hand applies fundal pressure to fix the head in the pelvis. If the operator is unable to accomplish rotation in this fashion, the middle and index fingers of the right hand are inserted into the vagina behind the ear to the posterior or left parietal bone. Rotation to an OA is performed with a lifting motion. If this is successful, the fingers remain in the vagina to act as a splint against the left parietal bone so that forceps may be applied. The left hand then aids by applying fundal pressure.

A modification of this technic is the simultaneous use of the fingers of the left hand to exert downward pressure on the right frontal area as the right-hand fingers elevate the left parietal area to induce rotation. Once rotation is accomplished, the right hand remains in the vagina to act as a splint so that forceps may be applied.

Should this maneuver fail, the right hand is introduced into the posterior segment of the pelvis with the palm up. The thumb applies gentle pressure on the sinciput to increase flexion. All force applied is equally distributed through all four fingers. Rotation is accomplished by a counterclockwise turn of the hand. Slight elevation of the head into a more spacious plane of the pelvis may be necessary. One of the inherent dangers of this technic, however, is the increased difficulty of forceps application and traction at a higher pelvic station.

For an ROT, the hands are reversed to perform manual rotation.

INSTRUMENTAL PROCEDURES

The proper and accurate application of forceps to a transverse arrest is probably the most difficult of all forceps operations. Since the etiology varies, there is no single forceps with which to manage the problem. When one is dealing with a simple transverse position due to conduction anesthesia, delivery can be accomplished with a conventional instrument. In a true transverse arrest which warrants rotation prior to extraction, the Kielland forceps offers unique advantages. The Barton forceps is the only instrument capable of safely applying traction to a transverse arrest without rotation; it is the instrument of choice for delivery of a transverse in a flat pelvis. The K-B forceps offers the advantages of the Barton forceps for application and the Kielland for rotation.

Two cardinal principles are fundamental to the use of forceps for a transverse arrest. Since the anterior segment of the pelvis is limited by the pubic rami, it is the least spacious. Hence, the anterior branch must be applied first. This avoids compromising the available space by lifting the head with the application of the posterior branch. The problem of asynclytism also demands special care. To achieve an accurate cephalic application in such cases, the forceps must have a sliding lock. If conventional forceps are applied to an asynclytic head, it is impossible to obtain a true cephalic application and then lock the branches.

Conventional Forceps

Conventional forceps are acceptable for the management of a synclytic transverse head which has not undergone extensive molding. Since 90° rotation must be accomplished, forceps with long overlapping shanks are most desirable. Forceps with parallel shanks tend to produce overstretching of the maternal tissues upon rotation. The Tucker-McLane forceps adequately fulfills the need. If the operator prefers an instrument with a sliding lock, Luikart's forceps is the one of choice. The solid or pseudofenestrated blades of these instruments also

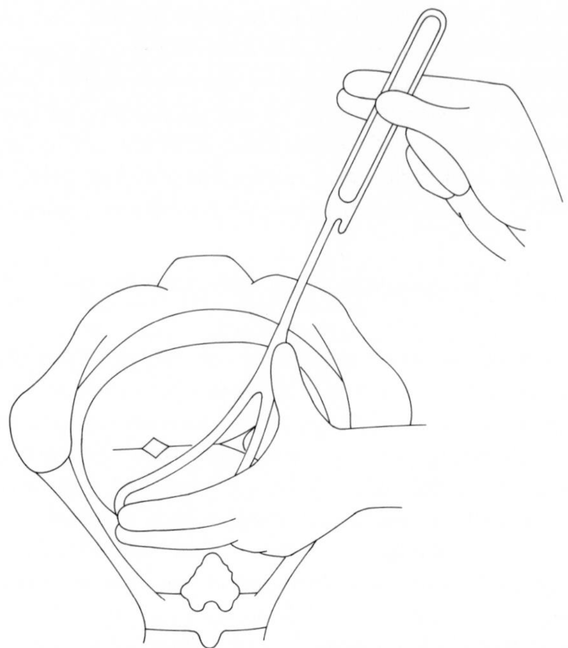

Fig. 9-1. Posterolateral insertion of anterior (*right*) branch, LOT.

eliminate the problem of hooking the blade over an ear or other points of obstruction.

For an LOT, the right or anterior branch is inserted and applied first. The handle is oriented toward the left maternal groin by the right hand so that the toe of the blade is directed toward the right posterior pelvic quadrant (Fig. 9-1). As the handle descends in its sweeping arc, the pelvic curve carries the blade—protected by the left hand in the vagina—into the pelvis and around the left frontal bone. The blade is now wandered around the face until it achieves its proper position in front of the right ear and over the right malarparietal area. Wandering is accomplished by controlling the handle with the right hand while the left index finger elevates the shank and assists the blade to curve around the face to its ultimate destination. Completion of the application brings the handle below the horizontal plane and close to the midline (Fig. 9-2).

The left or posterior branch is now inserted and applied (Fig. 9-3). The handle is controlled with the left hand while the right hand is inserted into the vagina. By orienting the handle to the left of the midline, the blade can be guided to the left of the other branch and along the hollow of the sacrum. If this branch is inserted on the right

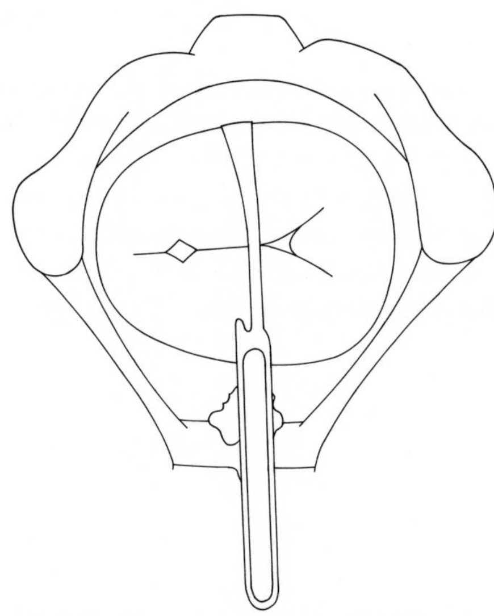

Fig. 9-2. Application of anterior (*right*) branch, LOT.

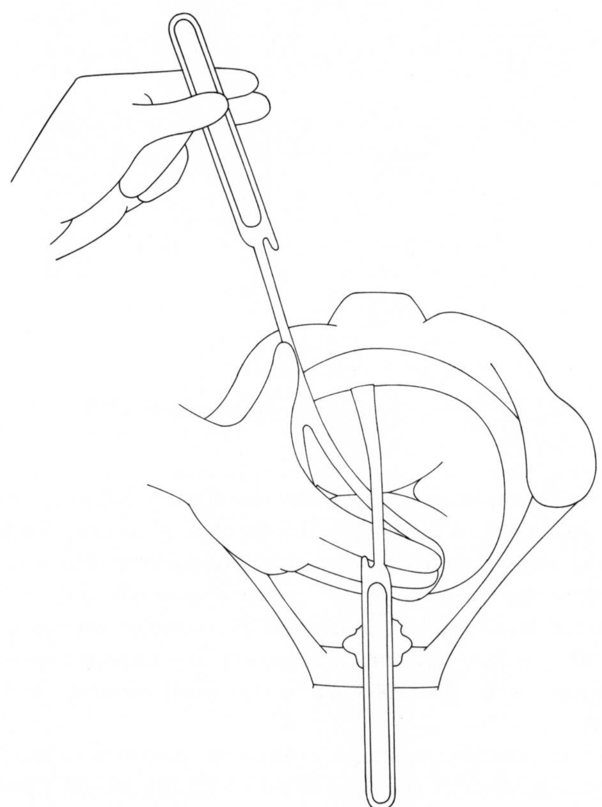

Fig. 9-3. Insertion of posterior (*left*) branch, LOT.

side, recrossing of the handles is necessary for articulation. Care must be taken to avoid undue force of insertion or the posterior vaginal wall and rectum will be damaged. When the level of proper application is reached, the handle will remain above the horizontal plane.

The branches are locked and the application secured and checked against the landmarks of the fetal skull. Flexion of the head is increased by moving the handles directly to the left in the horizontal plane.

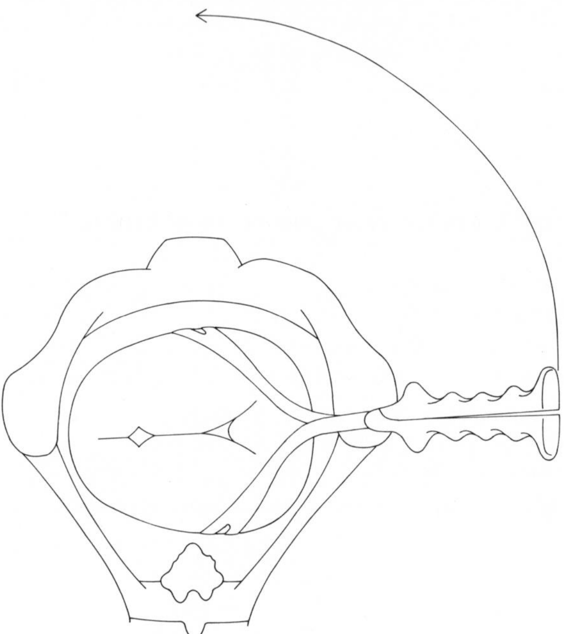

Fig. 9-4. Forceps application and rotation, LOT.

The lock should now be disengaged and the application of the branches adjusted if necessary. Once again the forceps is locked. Rotation is performed by sweeping the handles counterclockwise in a wide arc of 90° until they are parallel to the pubic symphysis (Fig. 9-4). The position of the fetal head is now checked to make certain that the sagittal suture is in the midline. If necessary, the forceps may again be adjusted. Traction is accomplished in the usual manner in the axis of the pelvis.

Resistance to rotation in simple transverse positions is usually due to persistent extension of the fetal head or failure of the operator to rotate the handles through a wide arc. With a true arrest which necessitates elevation of the head to a higher pelvic plane for rotation, it is probably wise to use a special instrument such as the Kielland.

For an ROT, the technic is reversed. First, the left or anterior blade is inserted, wandered, and applied. The right or posterior blade is then applied. One basic variation for right-sided positions is that the branches must be crossed in order to achieve proper locking. Crossing is facilitated by pushing one handle up and the other down. Flexion, rotation, and extraction are then performed. The operator usually will find more blade adjustments necessary in right-sided positions.

Rotation of a transverse vertex can be attempted by utilizing the posterior branch alone. Once inserted and applied, the branch is used as a simple vectis to elevate and rotate the occiput. This technic, however, fails to induce flexion of the head prior to rotation and is of limited value.

Barton Forceps

The Barton forceps is the only instrument with which traction can be safely applied to a transverse vertex in the transverse diameter of the pelvis. Hence, it is the forceps of choice for a transverse in a flat pelvis.[21] It is also indicated in the android type of pelvis when the operator desires to bring the head to a lower level for rotation. Whether or not it is used to complete the delivery in such cases, it is a most valuable forceps.

The technic of inserting and applying the Barton forceps is identical for either LOT or ROT. The hinged branch is the anterior one and is always applied first. It is introduced along the hollow of the sacrum (Fig. 9-5). Since the blades are symmetrical and quite thin, insertion

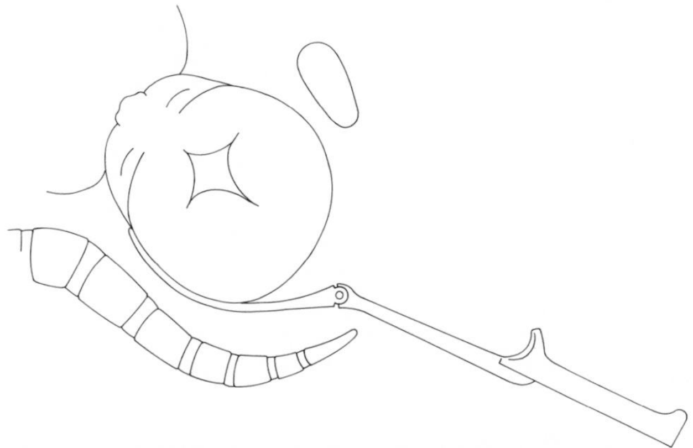

Fig. 9-5. Insertion of hinged branch, Barton forceps, LOT.

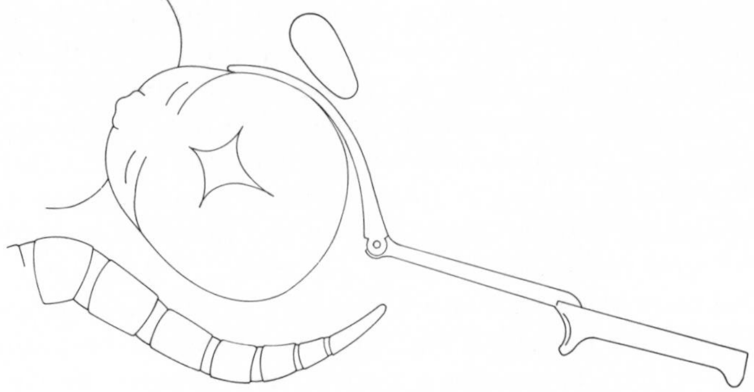

Fig. 9-6. Application of hinged branch, Barton forceps, LOT.

is usually easy to accomplish. The blade is now wandered over the occiput to its destination above the anterior parietal bone (Fig. 9-6). If resistance is met because of increased extension of the head, the blade can be wandered over the face. The easiest route is the one of choice. The shank and handle are now elevated and held by an assistant so that the posterior branch can be inserted. Care must be taken to avoid pinching the vaginal tissues in the hinge as the shank is elevated.

The posterior branch is now inserted along the hollow of the sacrum (Fig. 9-7). This is always done to the left of the anterior branch so that

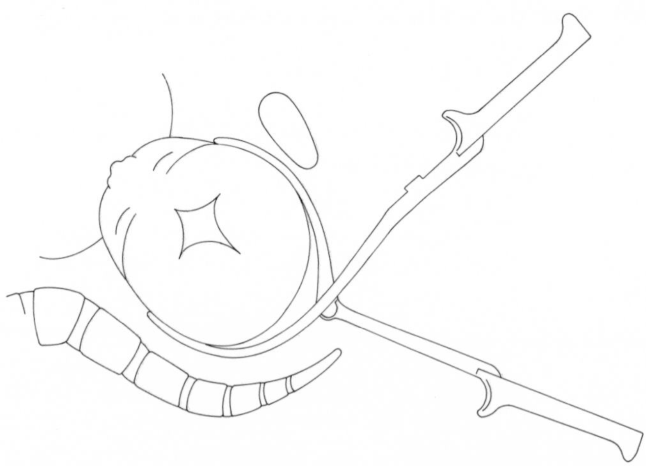

Fig. 9-7. Insertion of posterior branch, Barton forceps, LOT.

the branches will lock without having to be crossed. The handle is controlled by the right hand. The left middle and index fingers are inserted into the vagina and the shank controlled from below by the thumb. Occasionally, if the lower sacrum is anteflexed or particularly prominent, the head must be elevated to facilitate insertion of the posterior branch.

The branches are now engaged by the sliding lock on the posterior shank. The sliding lock allows this to be accomplished anywhere along the shank so that the blades can accommodate any asynclytism that is present.

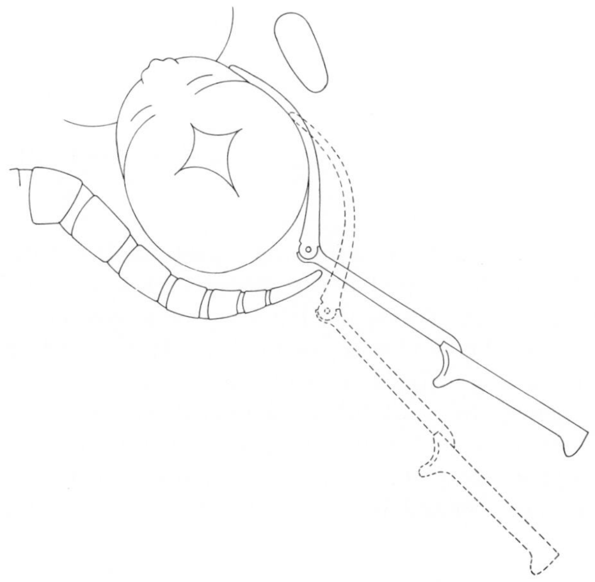

Fig. 9-8. Direct application of anterior branch, Barton forceps, LOT.

There is a second technic for the insertion of the anterior branch. When marked anterior parietal asynclytism is present, the hinged blade can be applied directly. The handle and shank are held in the midline beneath the perineum. The hinged blade is then inserted beneath the symphysis along the anterior parietal bone (Fig. 9-8). The operator must be certain that no residual anterior lip of cervix remains. If present, it must be elevated or pushed over the head to allow the blade to be inserted and applied.

Once the Barton forceps has been applied, traction is instituted.

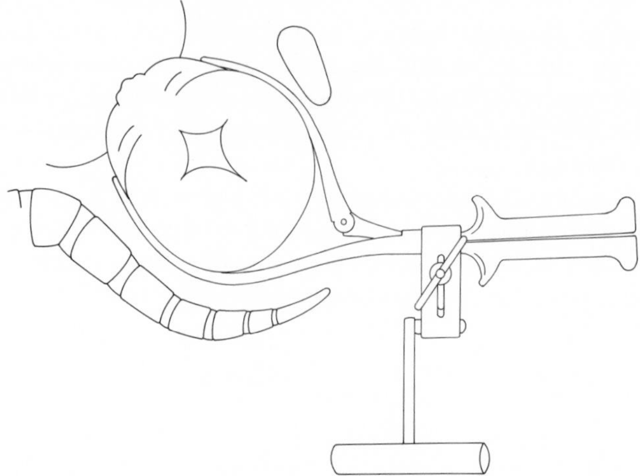

Fig. 9-9. Barton forceps application with traction handle.

This is performed either by adding the Barton traction handle to the shanks or by the Saxtorph-Pajot maneuver (Figs. 9-9 and 9-10). If manual traction is employed, the left hand depresses the shanks and the right elevates the handles in the midline. As the head descends in the transverse, any asynclytism present is gradually corrected.

In a flat pelvis, the head will frequently deliver in the transverse diameter. This is accomplished by simply continuing traction with the Barton forceps in the pelvic curve. If resistance is met at the outlet, however, the head should be rotated to the OA. The offset shanks

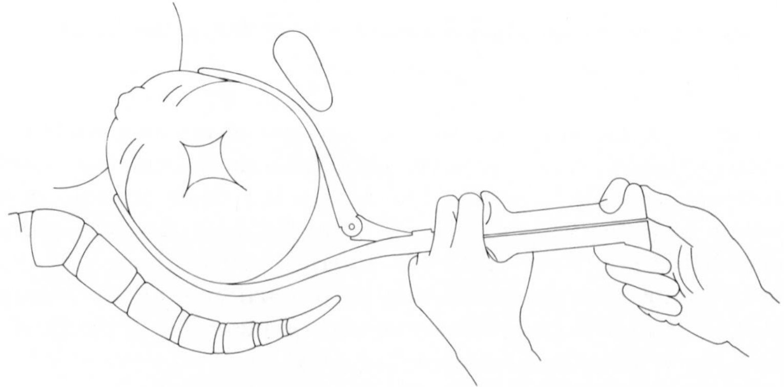

Fig. 9-10. Saxtorph-Pajot maneuver, Barton forceps.

and handles allow the forceps to perform this rotation when the handles are turned in a wide 90° arc to the horizontal. For an ROT, rotation is clockwise; for an LOT, counterclockwise. When rotation has been completed, the handles and shanks are approximately parallel to the horizontal but angled toward the maternal thigh in the direction of rotation. The operator may use the Barton forceps to complete the extraction or change to a conventional instrument. If the Barton is used following rotation, completion of the delivery is accomplished by applying direct traction to the crotch where the blades join the shanks. The operator must remember that in this position, the Barton forceps has no pelvic curve and increased depression of the handles is necessary.

With an android type of pelvis, the technic is different. The Barton forceps is still the instrument of choice for bringing the head down to a lower pelvic plane. Rotation, however, should be limited to 45° to reach an oblique diameter. Since this is the most spacious plane in this type of pelvis, it should be utilized for the extraction. In such cases it is advisable that a conventional forceps be applied for completion of the delivery in order to capitalize on its pelvic curve.

Kielland Forceps

The Kielland forceps and its modification (Kielland-Barton forceps) are the instruments of choice when one intends to manage a transverse arrest by rotation followed by traction. These forceps were designed for gynecoid and anthropoid pelves and are contraindicated in flat or android pelves.[26] Transverse arrests in a gynecoid or anthropoid pelvis may stem from prominent spines, failure of the powers to complete internal rotation, or from a borderline disproportion. These instruments, although no panacea, are the most effective rotators available for the management of these problems.

There are three technics available for the insertion and application of the Kielland forceps: the classic or *inversion* technic, the *wandering*, and the *direct*. These technics are based on the method used to insert and apply the anterior branch. The classic or inversion technic is the method originally described by Kielland and employs the intrauterine insertion of the anterior blade. Many who still favor the instrument have abandoned this technic because of its potential danger of trauma to the maternal tissues. The wandering technic seems safer, perhaps, but the length of the branches can make it an awkward procedure and hence difficult to control the toe of the blade. Direct application of the anterior branch is feasible only when there is marked anterior asynclytism. It has few advocates and is rarely employed.

Regardless of the method of insertion and application, and no matter how familiar or confident the operator feels with the Kielland instrument, there is one cardinal principle which must be followed. This principle is the external orientation of the forceps. The branches should be engaged and held outside the pelvis in the position they will finally assume when applied. The directional buttons must point toward the occiput. The operator should now grasp the anterior blade to be certain that he has the correct branch to begin the operation. The other branch should be put aside temporarily.

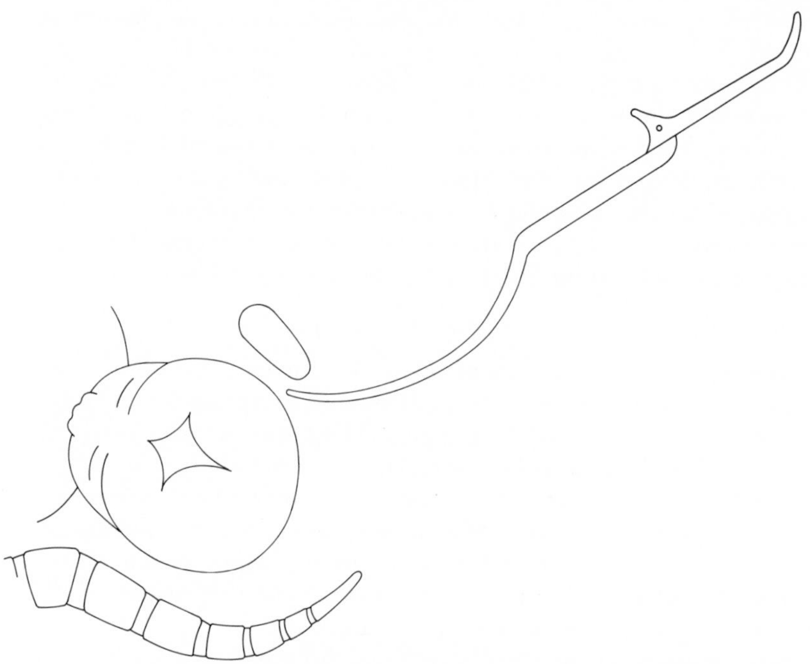

Fig. 9-11. Kielland forceps, inversion technic, orientation of anterior (*right*) branch, LOT.

For an LOT, the anterior branch is the right one. To insert and apply this branch by the *inversion* technic, the left middle and index fingers are first inserted under the symphysis, palmar surface up. If there is a residual lip of cervix present, it is elevated by the fingers to create a path between it and the anterior parietal bone for the blade to follow. The handle is controlled by the right hand. It is oriented in the midline and 45° above the horizontal so that the blade rests in the left palm, cephalic surface up. The directional marker on the finger grip is now pointed toward the anterior fontanelle since the branch is inverted (Fig. 9-11). As the handle is allowed to descend slowly in a vertical arc, the toe of the blade is guided over the finger tips and anterior parietal bone until the blade occupies the space in the lower uterine segment between the anterior shoulder and side of the head. At this point, the fenestration is no longer visible and the handle has dropped beneath the horizontal plane. The heel of the blade and the proximal shank are now over the anterior parietal bone

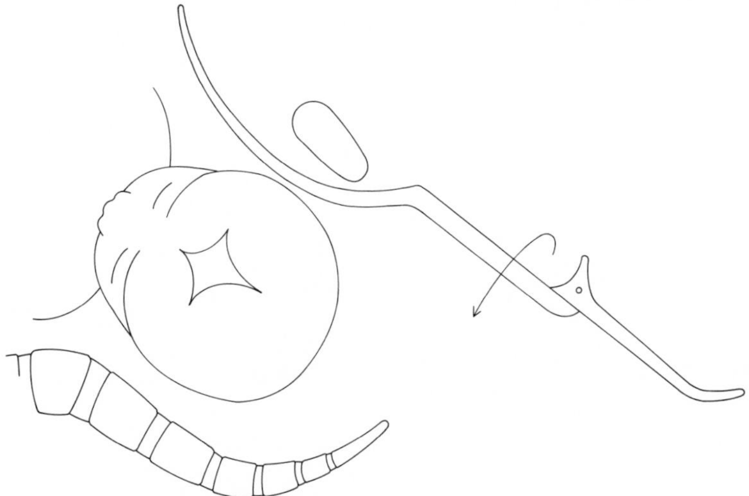

Fig. 9-12. Kielland forceps, inversion technic, insertion of anterior (*right*) branch, LOT.

(Fig. 9-12). One will usually observe a bulge on the lower abdominal wall due to the toe of the blade. The ultimate depth of insertion is related to the station of the head. The higher the station, the deeper the insertion and the lower the handle is beneath the horizontal plane. The maximum arc the handle will describe is 90°. Usually one is aware when the ultimate destination is reached as the proximal shank seems to drop over the parietal bone. Throughout this entire procedure, great care must be exercised. Any resistance encountered warrants cessation until the cause is determined. If necessary, this method of insertion is abandoned for another.

Once the insertion of the anterior branch has been completed and the blade has reached its proper level, it must be rotated 180° to complete the application. Rotation should be performed in a counter-clockwise direction toward the face. Advantage is then taken of the pelvic curve of the blade. Its gently curved surface provides less resistance than the more prominent toe and anterior rim of the blade. The handle is controlled with the right hand and the thumb is against the medial surface of the finger grip. Rotation is performed by a twisting motion of the wrist as if turning a door knob. The pivot point of rotation is in the axis of the shank. As the 180° arc of rotation is completed and the blade drops over the parietal bone in proper cephalic application, the operator is aware that the shank and handle have dropped to a lower level. The directional marker will now point toward the occiput (Fig. 9-13).

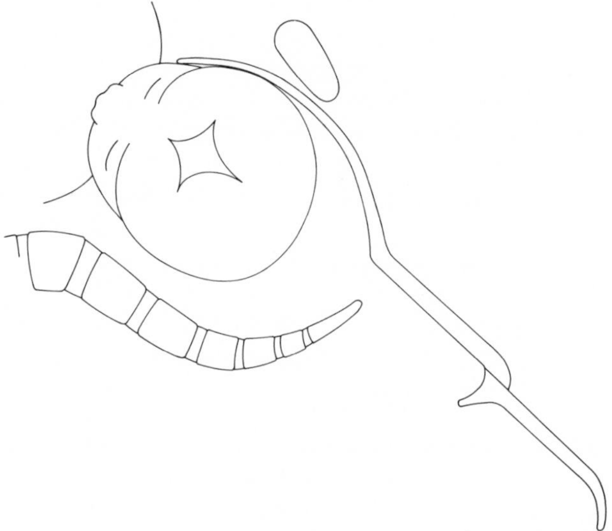

Fig. 9-13. Kielland forceps, inversion technic, application of anterior (*right*) branch, LOT.

Rotation of an inverted branch must be just as carefully performed as the insertion. If any resistance is encountered, rotation should cease. The operator should ascertain that the blade has been inserted inside the cervix and to the proper level. Occasionally, with a markedly extended head, rotation is easier to accomplish toward the occiput in a clockwise direction. This direction of rotation, however, should not be attempted unless rotation of the branch toward the face has been tried first. Although it can be safely performed, clockwise rotation does apply more pressure on the lower uterine wall because of the prominent toe of the blade.

There are many who prefer to apply the anterior branch of the Kielland forceps exclusively by *wandering* it into position. Advocates of this method believe it is less dangerous since it eliminates the intrauterine insertion and rotation of the anterior branch. One must remember, however, that the Kielland forceps is longer than most obstetric forceps, and therefore more difficult to control. Its increased length results in increased force and motion at the toe of the blade with manipulation of the handle. Application of the Kielland forceps by the wandering method can be just as traumatic as the inversion technic if not judiciously performed.

The branch is controlled and inserted as with any conventional instrument. Its handle should describe a wide lateral arc so that the blade will be inserted toward the right side of the pelvis. Wandering is performed clockwise around the face until the blade assumes its proper anterior position over the right parietal bone. If the head is well flexed and the space between the right frontal boss and pubic ramus reduced, difficulty will be encountered in wandering the blade about this point. It can be wandered counterclockwise over the occiput in such instances. Should the operator have this in mind prior to insertion, he must alter his technic. The handle should be held to the patient's right and beneath the horizontal plane with the directional marker toward the floor so that the blade will be oriented toward the left side of the pelvis. Once inserted, it is wandered upside down, around the occiput to its proper position. Care must be taken to avoid trauma to the anterior ear.

The least popular and most infrequently used technic of insertion of the anterior branch is the *direct* method. This should be performed only when there is marked anterior parietal asynclytism with the head approaching the outlet. In a direct application, the patient's buttocks should extend slightly over the edge of the delivery table. The branch is oriented in exactly the opposite direction of the inversion method. The handle is in the midline, controlled by the right hand, but pointed toward the floor. The middle and index fingers of the left hand are inserted palmar surface up to create a safe path for the blade. Any residual lip of cervix is elevated. The toe of the blade with its bevelled or cephalic surface downward is now put in contact with the anterior parietal bone. As the right hand directs the handle upward, the blade is guided under the symphysis and over the parietal bone. The insertion should be performed gently so that the blade can be directed toward the cheek in front of the ear. When performing a direct application of the anterior branch of the Kielland forceps, care must be taken to avoid contamination from the anus (Fig. 9-14).

To perform these methods of insertion of the anterior branch of the

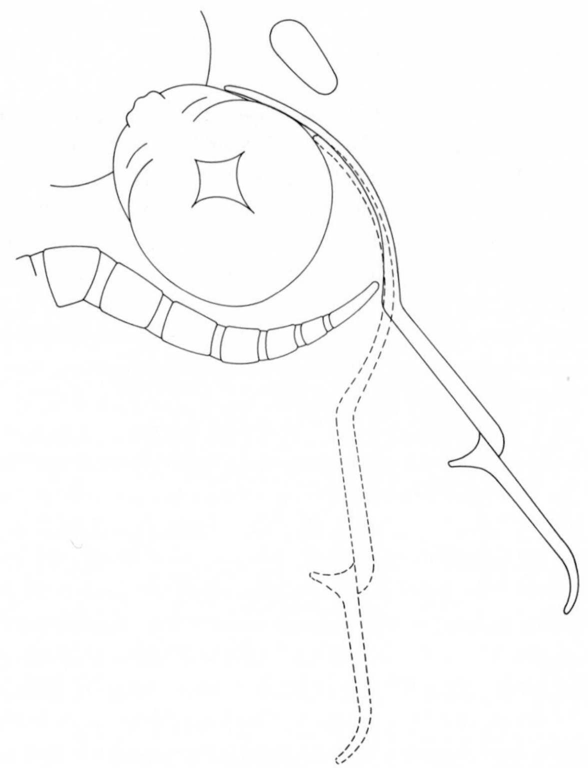

Fig. 9-14. Kielland forceps, direct application of anterior (*right*) branch, LOT.

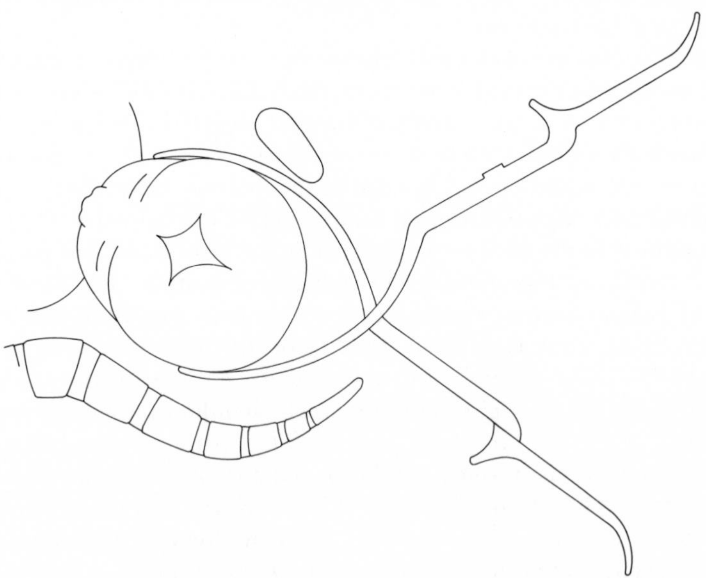

Fig. 9-15. Kielland forceps, insertion of posterior (*left*) branch, LOT.

Kielland forceps for an ROT instead of an LOT, the hands are reversed. The left hand controls the handle of the left branch, which is now the anterior one. The index and middle fingers of the right hand are the intravaginal guides to elevate any cervical rim and direct the course of the blade. If the inversion method of insertion is used, the branch is rotated clockwise toward the face.

The posterior branch of the Kielland forceps is always inserted along the hollow of the sacrum (Fig. 9-15). For an LOT, the left branch is the posterior one and is controlled by the left hand. The middle and index fingers of the right hand act as the intravaginal guide. They are inserted palmar surface up along the posterior vaginal wall. Once again, the operator must check for a residual lip of cervix. If present, the fingers are inserted between it and the posterior parietal bone. The handle is now held in the midline about 45° above the horizontal and to the left of the anterior branch to facilitate eventual locking. The blade, cephalic surface up, rests in the palm of the right hand. As the handle slowly descends, the blade is inserted along the posterior parietal bone. Since the cephalic curve of the Kielland blade is elongated and tapered, difficulty may be encountered from the increased curve of the sacrum. If the operator is certain that the resistance is not due to the cervix, he can ease the insertion by depressing the handle at intermittent intervals to allow the blade to hug the parietal bone. The ultimate destination of the posterior blade is dependent upon the degree of asynclytism which may be present. A deep

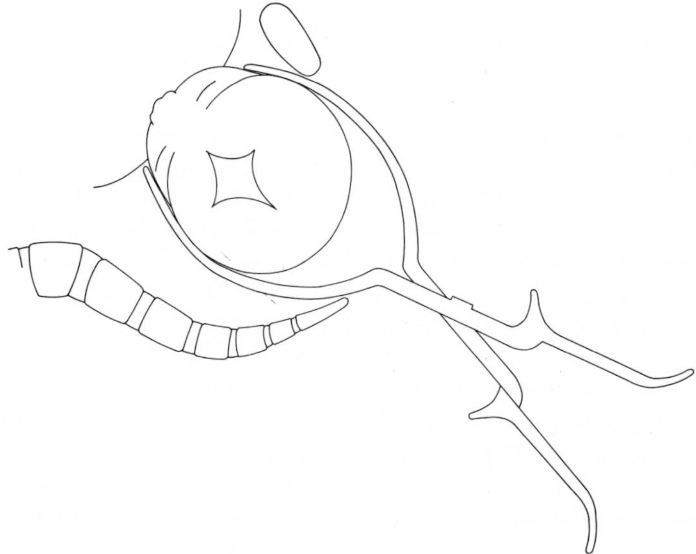

Fig. 9-16. Kielland forceps application, anterior parietal asynclytism, LOT.

insertion is required with anterior asynclytism, a shallow one with posterior asynclytism. When there is anterior parietal asynclytism present, the anterior branch will extend outward the farthest; and when there is posterior asynclytism, the posterior branch will extend the farthest (Figs. 9-16 and 9-17). Despite this variation, the branches are locked if the operator is confident he has achieved a biparietal application. The advantage of the sliding lock is now evident in that it allows articulation anywhere along the shank. The disparity between the branches will spontaneously correct itself when rotation has been completed. Occasionally an adjustment of the level of insertion of one or both branches is necessary to assure secure locking. The application of the branches is now checked with the landmarks of the fetal skull.

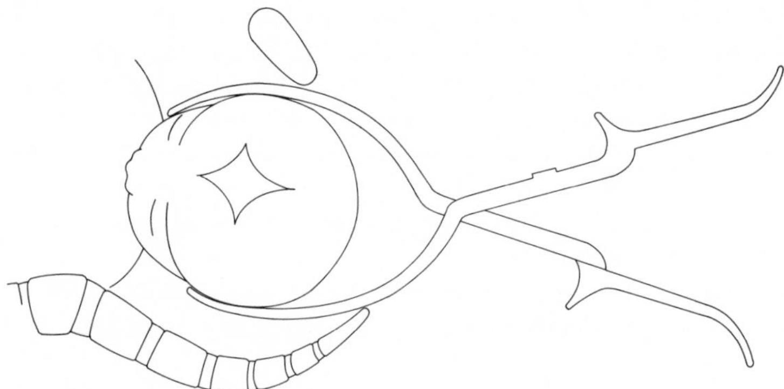

Fig. 9-17. Kielland forceps application, posterior parietal asynclytism, LOT.

Before initiating rotation, which is the primary function of the Kielland forceps, the operator should correct as much of the deflexion present as possible. This is accomplished by moving the handles horizontally toward the mother's right thigh and the fetal face. If necessary, the branches should be disengaged and the application adjusted. Since the pelvic curve of the Kielland blades is negated by the angulation of the shanks, rotation is performed in a very limited arc. This counterclockwise rotation is best accomplished by grasping the handles from below with the right hand. The thumb is against the left or upper finger guard and the index finger is hooked about the lower or right guard. Rotation is performed by pronating the hand (Fig. 9-18). Resistance to rotation may be due not only to persistent extension of the fetal head or its impaction against the ischial spines, but also to the operator's failure to perform rotation in the pelvic axis. The latter problem is corrected by depressing the handles to a lower level. Persistent extension or impaction against prominent spines may necessitate elevating the head to achieve rotation. As rotation is accomplished and the asynclytism corrects itself, the branches will assume a parallel alignment. When rotation has been completed, the handles should be depressed and slight downward traction applied in the pelvic axis to fix the head in the anterior posterior diameter.

For an ROT, the right branch is the posterior one. The hands are reversed, and the branch is inserted along the hollow of the sacrum to the left of the anterior branch to avoid crossing the handles for locking. Deflexion is corrected by moving the handles horizontally toward the left thigh, and rotation is performed clockwise.

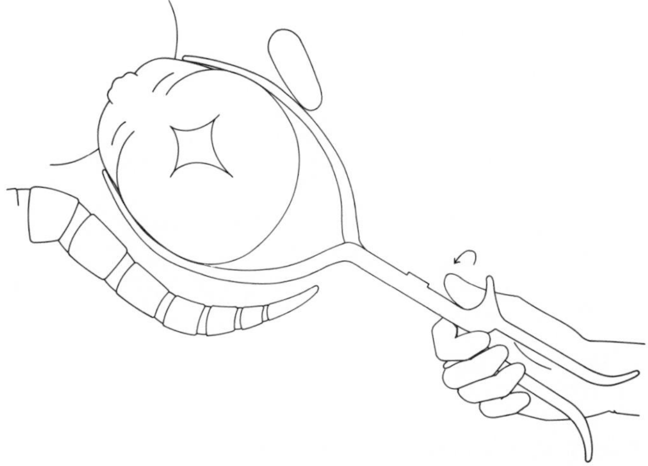

Fig. 9-18. Kielland forceps, rotation, LOT.

Once rotation from the transverse to the occiput anterior position has been completed, the Kielland forceps has fulfilled its primary function. The operator may prefer to change to a conventional forceps to complete the extraction. The Kielland forceps, however, will function adequately as a tractor if the technic of traction is adjusted to its construction. Traction with the Kielland instrument can be performed only with the vertex in the anteroposterior diameter. Traction should never be performed in the transverse plane since the bulging tapered blades will exert pressure against the bladder, urethra, and symphysis. The sequelae of such undue force are obvious.

Before instituting traction with the Kielland forceps, the application is rechecked. The handles are now lowered 45° below the horizontal. This compensates for the angulation of the shanks and blades and allows the pelvic curve of the blades to become functional. If traction is begun with the handles horizontal and then they are raised as the head is delivered, the pelvic curve of the blades will dig into the posterior vaginal walls and can create extensive sulcus lacerations.

An excellent way to achieve proper traction with the Kielland forceps is from the kneeling position. The operator's left knee is placed against the floor while the right one acts as a brace for the right arm.

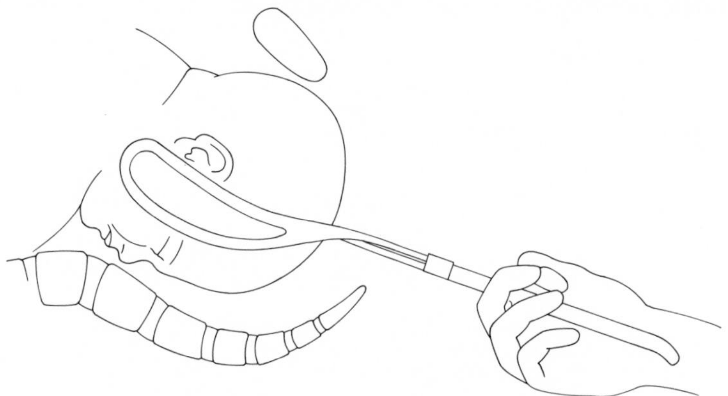

Fig. 9-19. Kielland forceps, traction following rotation.

The middle and index fingers of the right hand encircle the finger grips from below and the forearm extends downward to the right knee. Traction in this plane will compensate for the construction of the instrument and be in the proper axis of the pelvis (Fig. 9-19). Perineal distention due to the wide heels of the blades is relieved by a liberal posterolateral episiotomy. As the posterior fontanelle is delivered, the handles are gradually elevated toward the horizontal. It is wise to recheck the application at this point and make certain the shanks have not risen above the posterior fontanelle. If this has occurred, the branches should be unlocked, the handles depressed to the desired level, and the branches relocked. Traction and extension are then continued until the operator can perform the Ritgen maneuver.

The branches are removed in the usual manner. Resistance to removal may be due to a narrow pubic arch or to one of the blades being hooked over an ear. If necessary, the head can be delivered with one or both branches still applied.

Kielland-Barton (K-B) Forceps

The basic feature of this forceps is that it is inserted and applied as the Barton and used for rotation as the Kielland. For either right or left transverse positions of the occiput, the hinged branch is the anterior one just as with the Barton forceps. The lock of the hinged

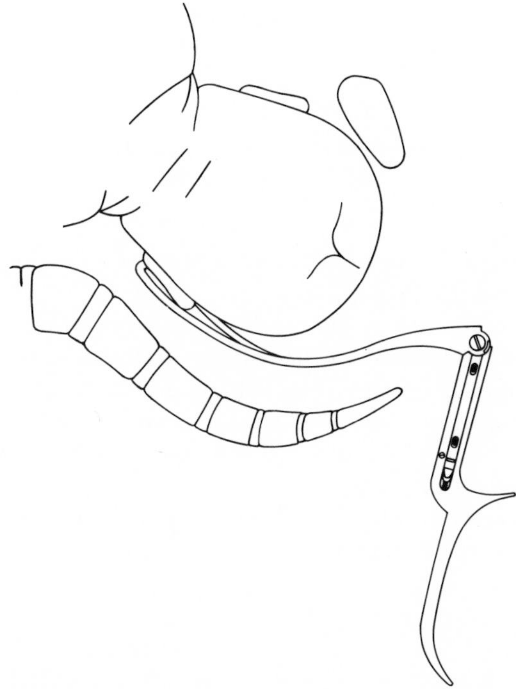

Fig. 9-20. Kielland-Barton forceps, posterior insertion of hinged branch, ROT.

branch is disengaged and the flail blade is gently introduced over the perineum along the hollow of the sacrum (Fig. 9-20). The blade is carefully wandered around and over the occiput until it assumes an anterior position beneath the symphysis. If resistance is met, the blade is wandered around the face. Wandering the blade over the occiput is usually easier if the vertex is well flexed; however, either route is acceptable, as with the Barton forceps. After the anterior blade has been applied, the lock remains disengaged so that the

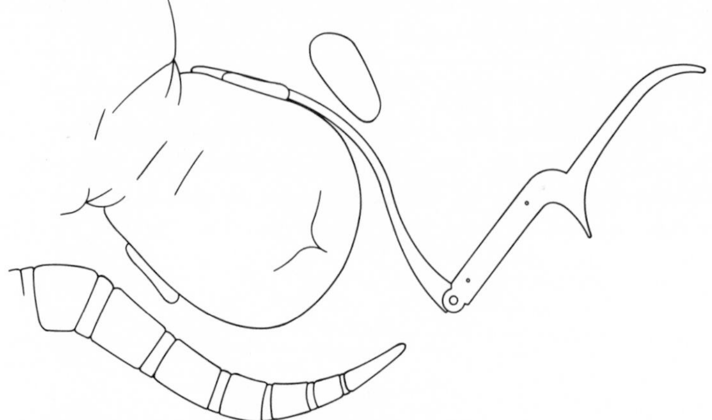

Fig. 9-21. Kielland-Barton forceps, application of anterior (hinged) branch, ROT.

handle and shank are out of the operator's path for the insertion of the posterior branch (Fig. 9-21).

The posterior branch is the rigid one and since the contour of its cephalic curve is identical to that of the Kielland, it is inserted and applied in a similar manner (Figs. 9-22 and 9-23). Because of its total length, this instrument, as the Kielland, possesses great leverage. Relatively little force applied at the end of the handle can inflict severe damage via the toe of the blade.

Once the posterior branch has been inserted and is in position, the anterior one is made rigid by dropping its handle. This allows the

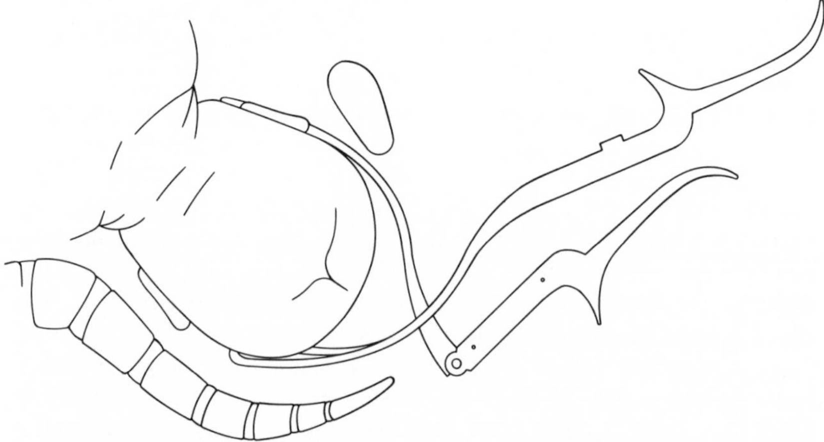

Fig. 9-22. Kielland-Barton forceps, insertion of posterior (rigid) branch, ROT.

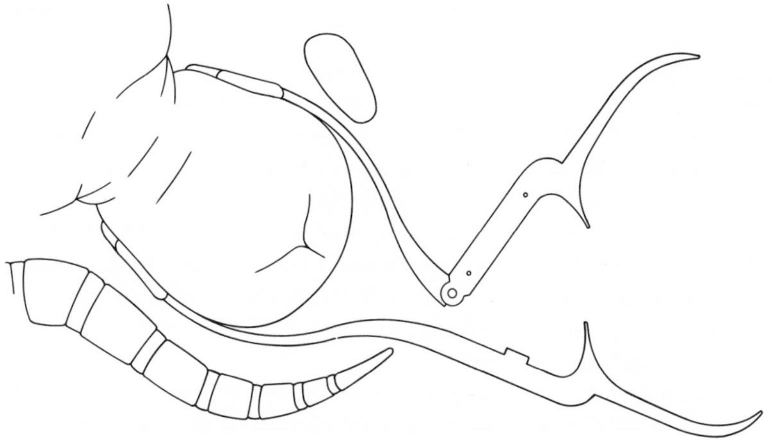

Fig. 9-23. Kielland-Barton forceps, application of posterior (rigid) branch, ROT.

spring lock to fix in place and the sliding lock of the shanks to engage. The operator now checks the accuracy of his forceps application. Since most transverse arrests are asynclytic, the shanks and handles, although parallel, will appear uneven in length as with the Kielland. When there is anterior parietal asynclytism, the anterior branch will extend outward the farthest; and when there is posterior asynclytism, the posterior branch will extend the farthest.

Occasionally, where there is marked anterior asynclytism, the anterior blade can be inserted directly over the anterior parietal bone (Fig. 9-24). A minimum of force should be used since the blade will

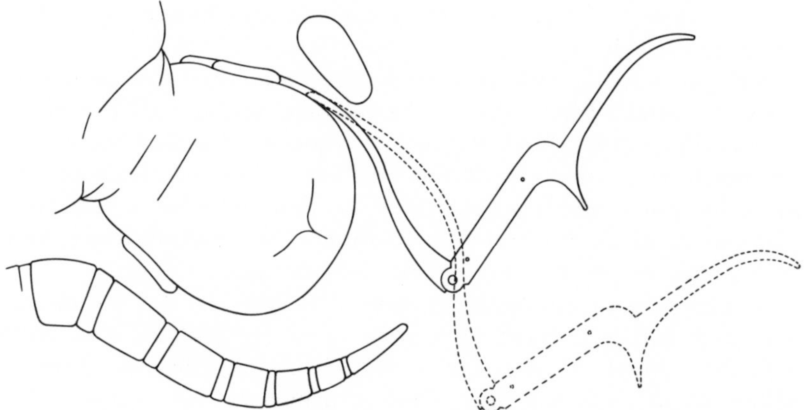

Fig. 9-24. Kielland-Barton forceps, direct application of anterior (hinged) branch, ROT.

follow the contour of the fetal head. The only obstruction one should encounter is the ear, and gentle lateral manipulation will allow the blade to slip by. When this type of application is attempted, the patient's buttocks should be at the very edge of the table and care should be exercised to avoid contamination from the rectum.

Once the forceps is applied, the first step is to check for the degree of flexion of the fetal head. Extension of the vertex is corrected by moving the handles of the forceps horizontally toward the face. The branches should then be disengaged, returned to a position over the parietal bones, and relocked.

In order to assure the application of minimal force with rotation, the handles should be turned as with the Kielland. Since the blades are symmetrical and do not possess a pelvic curve, the arc of rotation of the handles is kept to a minimum. Resistance to rotation may require elevation of the head into a larger diameter of the pelvis. As rotation is accomplished and the sagittal suture approaches the midline, the branches assume an even, parallel position. Slight traction is now employed in a 45° angle toward the floor to assure fixation of the vertex in the OA position.

If the operator desires to deliver the infant with this instrument, traction must be continued at a 45° angle as with the Kielland forceps. As the occiput fixes beneath the symphysis and the head begins to extend, the handles of the forceps are gently raised to the horizontal. This avoids the traumatic digging of the toes of the blades into the vaginal sulci. One must remember that this instrument, as the Kielland, has a wide diameter between the heels of the blades and a liberal episiotomy is usually warranted.

If the operator prefers, the K-B forceps can be removed once rotation has been accomplished and a conventional forceps applied to complete the delivery.

Perhaps the most important concept regarding the management of transverse arrests from below is the individuality of each procedure. The Barton forceps, for instance, is unique in its ability to provide traction to a transverse head as a transverse. The indication for the use of this instrument is the absolute contraindication for the Kielland. The latter's primary function is rotation. These instruments cannot be expected to perform more than they were intended to.

Duplicity does exist, however, in that the operator has a choice of maneuver and instrument in selected cases. He should be as adept with the manual technics as with instrumental rotation. He must be willing to abandon any instrument or maneuver if he suspects that it may lead to undue force. To rely exclusively on one instrument or procedure indicates failure to fully comprehend the various etiologies of transverse arrests and the obstetric forceps designed to manage them.

*

Chapter Ten

*

Occiput Posterior Positions

Occiput posterior arrest of the fetal head is the most frequent major complication which can be amenable to forceps delivery. It, too, has prompted innumerable reviews and the innovation of many special technics. One must remember, however, that not only will some occiput posterior positions deliver spontaneously, but others frequently can be managed with outlet forceps. (*See* Chapter 7.) The residual arrests are those which have ceased to make progress. Two hours of observation in the nullipara and one hour in the multipara after complete cervical dilatation are considered adequate indication for intervention. This approach will aid in reducing the increased fetal and maternal morbidity and mortality which are associated with occiput posterior arrests. Here again, the operator must determine whether or not cesarean section is the procedure of choice before attempting either a major vaginal maneuver or forceps operation.

Occiput posterior positions constitute 4–5 per cent of all vaginal deliveries. The ROP position is 3–5 times more frequent than LOP. The rectosigmoid and the dextrorotation of the uterus are believed to be the factors which contribute to this discrepancy.

Occiput posterior positions and arrests can occur in any pelvis with a reduced transverse diameter. In an anthropoid pelvis, a posterior may be the normal mechanism of labor. Other pelvic factors which may cause occiput posterior orientation of the fetal head are prominent ischial spines and reduced capacity of the forepelvis. Increased convergence of the lateral pelvic walls or a straight sacrum may cause the fetal head to descend as a posterior in one of the oblique diameters. Deflexion of the fetal head, late uterine inertia, and the premature use of conduction anesthesia also may lead to occiput posterior positions.

As with transverse arrests, a variety of manual and instrumental procedures are available for the management of the problem.

MANUAL ROTATION

The simplest manual procedure which can be attempted to induce a posterior position to undergo anterior rotation is the Hodge maneuver. As with transverse arrests, this must be attempted while there are effective uterine contractions.

The most frequently employed method of manual rotation for posterior positions, however, is the one described by Willson in his *Atlas of Obstetric Technic.*[109] For an ROP, the palm of the left hand is placed beneath the occpiut so that the thumb and fingers are over the opposite parietal bones. Flexion of the head is encouraged by pressure at the occiput. Gentle but continuous pressure is then applied to the head by pronating the forearm, until the occiput reaches an anterior position. Elevation of the head during this procedure should be avoided or kept to a minimum. During this maneuver, the right hand applies external pressure to the fetal shoulders to assist rotation of the body. Once manual rotation is completed, the head should be held in place until the forceps is applied. This will prevent the head from rotating back to the posterior position. For an LOP, the hands of the operator are reversed.

The Holland method is an alternative technic of manual rotation. For an ROP, the right hand is employed with the palmar surface over the forehead and face. Following an attempt to flex the head, rotation is accomplished by supination of the forearm.

If manual rotation cannot be accomplished beyond the transverse plane, the operator may apply the forceps as to a transverse arrest.

The Pomeroy maneuver[26] is the most complex of all manual technics. It is now primarily of historic interest. Briefly it can be described as elevating the head in the pelvis, grasping the impinged posterior shoulder, and rotating the infant 180°. To accomplish this for an ROP, the operator employs his left hand. It is placed beneath the occiput, palmar surface up so that the head can be lifted into a higher pelvic plane. Once the vaginal hand has been properly placed, the attendant turns his back to the patient—a position that is necessary if adequate leverage is to be gained for rotation. Following elevation of the head, the hand is inserted deeper into the pelvic canal so that the impinging posterior shoulder can be grasped between the index and middle fingers. Frequently it becomes necessary for the operator to kneel (still with his back to the patient) in order to properly grasp the shoulder. Rotation is again performed by pronation of the

Ortho Pharmaceutical Corporation

RARITAN • NEW JERSEY 08869

In our continuing search for better methods of contraception, we at Ortho have never forgotten that the historic purpose of conception control has been to ensure that procreation is planned, not left to chance.

We have always emphasized the positive aspects of contraception in the conviction that its ultimate purpose is to improve the quality of life--for mother and child.

Just as a woman deserves safe, effective means of preventing conception--when that is her goal--she deserves the best obstetric care when she decides to become pregnant. Accordingly, we feel that any contribution we can make to good obstetric technic is as important as are our efforts to improve contraceptive practice.

We therefore take pleasure in presenting you with this copy of Obstetric Forceps, by Leonard E. Laufe, M.D. It is an enlightening account of the history and uses of this simple yet versatile instrument. We hope it will be of value to you in your future practice.

Sincerely,

Ortho Pharmaceutical Corporation

forearm. As this is being accomplished, the operator turns and faces the patient. Rotation should be a full 180°, i.e., ROP to LOA. Rotation is enhanced by exerting pressure to the anterior shoulder with the external hand. Once completed, fundal pressure is applied to assist the head to return to a lower pelvic plane.

The patient must first be deeply anesthetized before the Pomeroy maneuver can be performed. This factor and the inherent danger of prolapse of the cord are the reasons that the procedure has been abandoned by most obstetricians.

An interesting and unique maneuver which may eliminate the need for manual or forceps rotation of a posterior position is the Puddicombe procedure. In a limited series of 27 cases of posterior position, Puddicombe was able to induce anterior rotation by placing his patients on their knees and elbows in a crawl position. In a matter of moments, spontaneous rotation occurred with subsequent improvement in the quality of the labor. Despite the simplicity of this procedure, it has yet to achieve great popularity.

INSTRUMENTAL PROCEDURES

There is a greater choice of instruments and procedures for the management of occiput posterior positions than for any other type of delivery. The alternatives can be categorized, however, into three major groups: extraction of the posterior position as a posterior; rotation to an anterior position by special maneuvers with conventional forceps; and rotation with special instruments.[15,16,19,20,50] Too frequently the obstetrician tends to limit management of the problem to a single technic or instrument. This is unfortunate, since a change in technic of rotation or choice of forceps may simplify what appears to be a difficult problem.

Proper evaluation of each case is the only means of determining what is necessary to successfully conclude the delivery. X-ray pelvimetry can give the attendant the assurance that no disproportion exists, or can supply the information which prevents a traumatic forceps delivery. Careful clinical appraisal of the pelvis can influence the choice of maneuver or forceps. Other pertinent factors which influence the type and time of intervention are the physical status of the mother and infant, the duration of labor, parity, and the degree of molding of the fetal head.

Delivery of a Posterior as a Posterior

There are an appreciable number of posterior positions which do not reach the pelvic floor and yet are still best delivered as posteriors. This is particularly true in patients with a marked anthropoid pelvis. If the labor is prolonged and the mother begins to show signs of exhaustion, the operator may elect to extract the infant before the occiput reaches the perineum. Perineal bulging or crowning with posterior positions is not necessarily indicative that outlet forceps can be applied. Because of the pronounced molding of a posterior vertex, particularly in a primipara, the caput will appear at the introitus long before the perineal floor has been reached by the occiput.

If such a forceps delivery is undertaken, the operator must be cognizant that he will be performing a midforceps procedure. Choice of forceps should be restricted to those with long tapered blades to accommodate the accentuated molding. The forceps are applied in the same manner as outlet forceps to a posterior position, the toes of the blades curving away from the ears and toward the mouth. Great care must be taken with the application, since the molding and edema may make some of the landmarks of the fetal skull difficult to identify.

Rotation to the direct occiput posterior from an ROP to LOP position is usually required prior to traction. It is performed by slightly depressing the handles through an arc in the desired direction. Once the anteroposterior plane has been reached, the cardinal landmarks are checked again in order to determine that slippage of the blades has not occurred.

Traction must be employed at an increased angle to compensate for the higher pelvic station and to allow the sinciput to pass beneath the pubic arch. A liberal posterolateral episiotomy is usually indicated to compensate for the increased perineal distention by the occiput and parietal bosses. Trial traction of a posterior arrest as a posterior prior to a contemplated rotation is worthwhile. Frequently the operator will be rewarded by an easier delivery than anticipated.

The Simpson forceps with the Bill traction handle or one of the axis-traction modifications of the Simpson is well suited for the midforceps extraction of a posterior as a posterior. An ideal instrument, however, is the Hawks-Dennen forceps with its tapered fenestrated blades and inherent axis-traction (*see* Fig. 7-6).

Rotary Maneuvers

The Scanzoni maneuver is perhaps the best known, and most modified, of all forceps procedures. Although Smellie was the first to recommend the use of forceps as an aid to rotation, Scanzoni was the first to make instrumental rotation the primary feature of a forceps operation. In order to appreciate the ultimate modifications of Scanzoni's technic, it is pertinent to review his original report. The following quotation is from Reddoch's translation[80]:

The head stands with the forehead turned toward the front and left, so that the sagittal suture passes in the right oblique diameter; the left blade is applied in front of the left sacroiliac synchrondrosis, the right behind the right obturator foramen; with this the transverse diameter of the forceps is placed in the left oblique diameter of the pelvis, their concave edges and tips are turned to the anterior circumference of the left lateral hemisphere of the pelvis, and so also with the forehead. An eighth of a circle is now described with the instrument, directed from left to right, whereby its right blade comes to rest under the symphysis, and the left in the hollow of the sacrum; and in this way, the head is rotated, the earlier standing forehead is moved to the middle of the left lateral wall of the pelvis and the sagittal suture is placed parallel with the transverse diameter of the pelvis.

Now both blades of the forceps are removed, and again applied, so that the left blade comes to lie behind the left obturator foramen, the right in front of the right sacroiliac ligament, whereupon by the next rotation the occiput is brought completely under the pubic arch.

It wasn't long before most obstetricians who were employing Scanzoni's maneuver extended the rotation to 90° or 135° so the occiput would reach an anterior position. At this point, the second application of the forceps was made to complete the extraction. This modification is the one most commonly employed today. An ROP is considered as an LOA and the branches of the forceps are inserted and applied accordingly. Thus the left blade is the posterior one and is applied first. The right blade is then inserted, wandered into place, and the branches articulated. With proper application the posterior fontanelle will be below the plane of the shanks. The head is flexed by elevating the handles in the right oblique diameter of the pelvis. Following flexion, it may be necessary to disarticulate the branches, adjust the application, and relock the branches. The handles are then rotated clockwise through a wide arc (Fig. 10-1). This is necessary to maintain the blades in the center of the pelvis (Fig. 3-5) and to avoid injury to the soft tissues. If resistance to rotation is encountered, the operator must desist from rotation until the problem is reevaluated. If the head is tightly wedged into the pelvis, elevating it to a higher station will assist rotation.

Once rotation has been completed, the handles are pulled downward over the perineum to assist the head to fix in its new position, the branches are unlocked, removed, reinverted, and reapplied. Removal of each branch is performed by directing its handle downward and outward. The forceps is now reapplied in a classic fashion and the extraction completed.

There are a variety of modifications of this technic which have been developed to prevent the head from rotating back to its original position. One of the most popular is the retention of one blade as a "splint." Instead of removing both branches following rotation of an

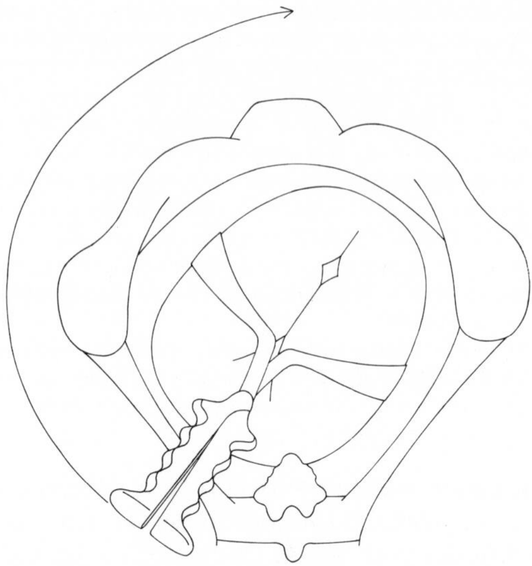

Fig. 10-1. ROP, Tucker-McLane forceps, Scanzoni maneuver, wide rotary arc.

ROP to an OA, the left branch—which is now on the right side of the pelvis—is allowed to remain in place. It acts as a splint until the right branch is removed and reinserted. In order for this to be accomplished, the right blade must be inserted between the left blade and the baby's head. A variation of this technic is to employ a second pair of forceps for the second application.[91]

Another commonly employed modification which has been popularized by King, Herring, and King is the intravaginal wandering of one blade from one side to the other. The wandered branch assumes its proper relationship to the occiput while splinting the anterior position.

There are also variations of the Scanzoni maneuver related to the extraction. The most popular one is the use of the Bill traction handle. Kutcipal reports that delivery can be accomplished with the forceps in the inverted position. He emphasizes, however, that it is mandatory for the operator to direct traction markedly downward over the perineum to properly impinge the occiput under the symphysis.

One of the more ingenious and practical variations of the Scanzoni procedure is that practiced by Williams and Cosgrove, as well as others.[1] They advocate applying the forceps in an inverted manner in relation to the pelvis. With this technic, the blades are properly applied to the fetal head. Following rotation, the forceps not only maintains a proper relationship to the head but is properly oriented to the pelvis. There is no need, therefore, to remove and reapply the forceps prior to instituting traction.

In the "inverted" Scanzoni maneuver, the operator's first step is to externally orient the forceps. For an ROP, the forceps is held as for an LOA and then turned upside down. This places the left handle in the right hand and the right handle in the left. The posterior branch is applied first. Since the pelvic curve is reversed, the blades must be inserted from below. The handle of the inverted right or posterior

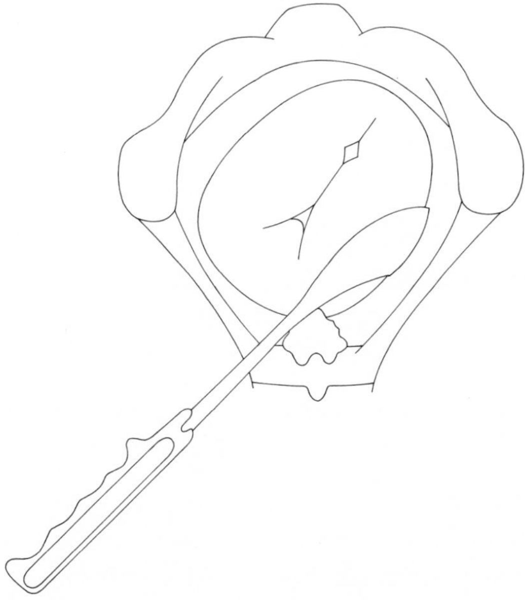

Fig. 10-2. ROP, Tucker-McLane forceps, insertion posterior (*right*) branch, inverted Scanzoni maneuver.

branch is held 45° below the horizontal and toward the right maternal thigh (Fig. 10-2). The toe of the blade is inserted along the left side of the vagina, the tissues being protected by the fingers of the right hand. The blade is directed about the right parietal boss as the handle describes an upward arc toward the midline. The critical aspect of the insertion is the need to prevent the pelvic curve of the blade from traumatizing the maternal tissues.

The anterior or inverted left branch is now inserted and applied in a similar manner, but the blade is directed more toward the an-

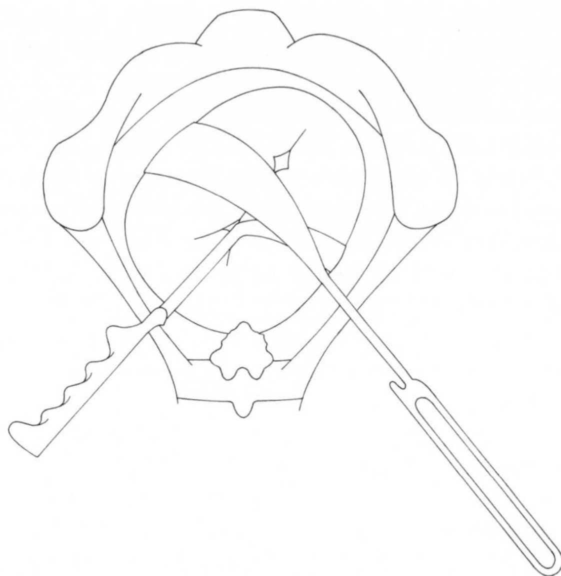

Fig. 10-3. ROP, Tucker-McLane forceps, insertion anterior (*left*) branch, inverted Scanzoni maneuver.

terior half of the right pelvic wall (Fig. 10-3). The application of each branch is checked, adjusted if necessary, and then the forceps is locked. With the forceps properly applied to an ROP, the anterior fontanelle will be above the inverted shanks and the posterior fontanelle one finger's breadth below. The handles should point downward and be in line with the right oblique diameter of the pelvis (Fig. 10-4).

Flexion of the head is encouraged by elevating the handles in the right oblique plane and rotation is performed by a wide clockwise arc with the handles. Once rotation has been completed and the head has achieved an occiput anterior position, the application is rechecked and any necessary adjustments made. Traction is now instituted and the extraction completed.

For an LOP, the branches are reversed.

The inverted Scanzoni maneuver is surprisingly easy to perform in a multipara due to the previously stretched soft tissues. When performed in a primipara, great care must be taken with this procedure to avoid trauma to the maternal soft tissues.

The instrument which has achieved the greatest popularity for the performance of the Scanzoni maneuver or one of its modifications is

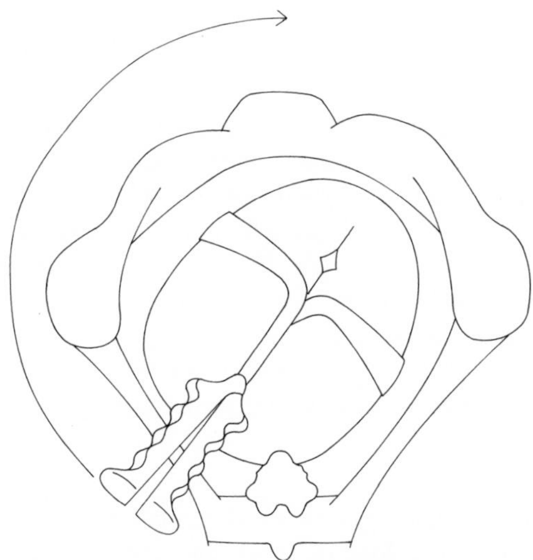

Fig. 10-4. ROP, Tucker-McLane forceps, application for inverted Scanzoni maneuver.

the Tucker-McLane forceps. The solid blades allow for easy insertion and wandering and the long overlapping shanks minimize distention of the introitus during rotation. Despite these advantages, some obstetricians prefer a Simpson-type instrument since the blades offer a better fit to the excessively molded head which is so frequent with posterior arrests.

There are a variety of other rotary maneuvers which have achieved limited degrees of popularity. Some are still practiced in the geographic area where they originated while others have gradually been replaced by other technics. One of the better known procedures, and yet infrequently practiced today, is the key-in-lock maneuver of DeLee.[23] Designed to mimic natural rotation and minimize trauma to the introitus, it is a series of gradual rotations (5–10° at a time) of a posterior position by multiple readjustments of the blades. Because of the increased number of manipulations, it has been replaced by other procedures.

Other rotary technics available for the management of the occiput posterior arrest employ a single branch. One branch can be used as a vectis or shoehorn to rotate the occiput to an anterior position. Maughan advocates a single branch of a fenestrated (De Wees) forceps over the anterior ear and rotating the head to a transverse position. The posterior branch is then applied, and rotation and extraction completed.

SPECIAL FORCEPS

Of all the special obstetric forceps, the Kielland has achieved greater popularity than any other for the management of occiput posterior arrests. Its preference is well deserved, for the Kielland is the best rotator. The K-B forceps, since it functions as the Kielland, also is suitable for these problems. And Barton forceps can be used for rotating a posterior position, but a second forceps application is usually required for the extraction. In addition, there is a group of special instruments with movable blades or shanks which have been designed to accomplish both rotation and extraction by a single application.[43,61,65]

Kielland Forceps

Since the directional markers of the Kielland must always point toward the occiput, the forceps is upside down when oriented for a posterior position. For an ROP, the shanks will be in the plane of the right oblique diameter of the pelvis, the markers will point toward the floor, and the pelvic curve of the blades will be inverted. The insertion and application of the blades should be accomplished by the wandering technic. Rarely is it necessary to apply the anterior blade by the inversion method, although this is preferred by some.

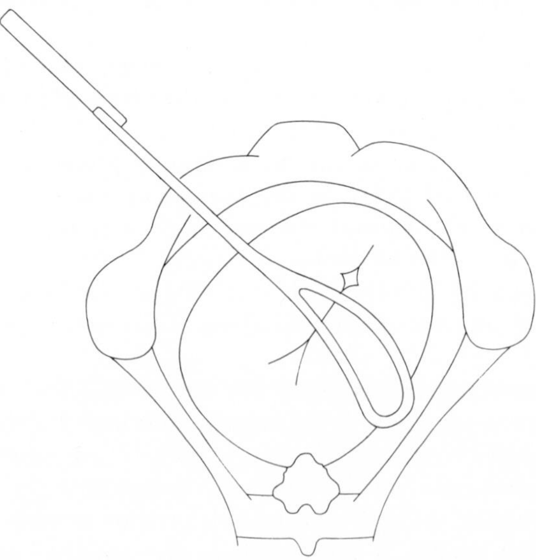

Fig. 10-5. ROP, Kielland forceps, insertion of posterior (*right*) branch.

When applied for an ROP, the right branch is the posterior one. It is inserted into the left posterior quadrant of the pelvis so that the cephalic curve of the blade is in apposition to the right side of the infant's head. Proper application can be easily accomplished by increasing the lateral angulation of the handle, which is controlled by the left hand (Fig. 10-5). The left or anterior branch is then inserted into the right posterior quadrant of the pelvis (Fig. 10-6). It must be carefully wandered over the occiput to its proper position. This is done by elevating the shank with the left index finger and depressing the handle with the right hand. Once both branches are properly applied, they are locked and the application is checked.

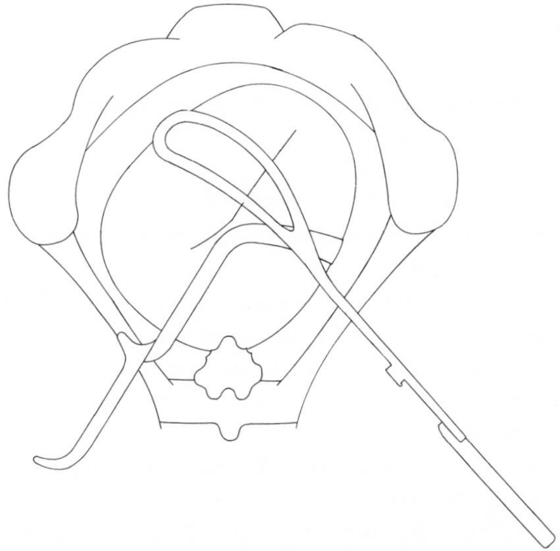

Figure 10-6. ROP, Kielland forceps, insertion of anterior (*left*) branch.

Any asynclytism present is corrected by adjusting the branches by traction until the finger grips are in the same place. The head is now flexed by elevating the handles, the branches adjusted if necessary, and rotation begun. Just as with transverse positions, rotation is performed through a narrow arc and best controlled with the thumb and index finger of the right hand (Fig. 10-7). For an ROP, clockwise rotation is carried out over an arc of 135°. If the head has been impacted into the pelvis, it may be necessary to elevate it to a higher station to accomplish rotation. Once rotation has been completed,

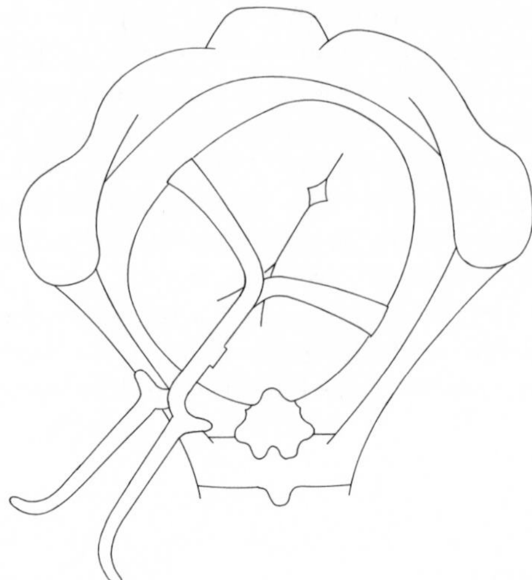

Fig. 10-7. ROP, Kielland forceps application.

downward traction will aid in fixing the head in the pelvis in its anterior position. The external hand frequently can be used to assist the shoulders in rotating.

The operator may elect to institute traction with the Kielland forceps, and this should be performed as previously described for transverse arrests. Some prefer, however, to remove the Kielland forceps once rotation has been accomplished and complete the delivery with a conventional instrument.

For an LOP, the branches are reversed, of course, and rotation is performed in a counterclockwise direction.

If used for a direct OP, the Kielland is best inserted from below the horizontal. In this technic, the inverted left branch is applied first, since it has the lock. This prevents having to recross the branches following insertion of the right one. As with the inverted Scanzoni maneuver, the handle of each branch should be 45° below the horizontal to initiate the insertion.

Kielland-Barton (K-B) Forceps

The K-B forceps is also well suited for the management of posterior arrests since its primary function is also rotation. Since the blades are absolutely symmetrical, they are not oriented to the fetal occiput with directional markers as are those of the Kielland forceps. The hinged branch becomes the posterior one for operative ease and is inserted first. Although insertion of this branch in a flail state allows for more sensitive control when wandering the blade, it can be inserted and wandered while rigid. Whether or not used in the hinged fashion, once the blade is applied the spring lock should be disengaged in order to keep the shank and handle out of the path of the rigid branch, which becomes the anterior one. This should be performed by inserting the blade into the appropriate posterior pelvic quadrant and wandering it into proper position.

If the position of the vertex is direct occiput posterior, the hinged branch is still applied initially as a matter of technical ease. Since the instrument is long, it is advantageous not to have the handle and shank of the first branch crossing the operative field. The spring lock is engaged following application of the second branch and the branches are then articulated. The accuracy of application is now checked and adjusted if necessary.

Flexion of the head is encouraged by elevating the handles toward the anterior fontanelle in a plane parallel to the sagittal suture. Rotation is accomplished as with the Kielland, i.e., the handles are turned with the thumb and forefinger as a key in a lock. The arc of rotation is kept to a minimum since there is no functional pelvic curve to the blades. Traction is also performed as with the Kielland forceps.

Barton Forceps

Although designed to apply traction to a transverse arrest in the transverse diameter of the pelvis, the Barton forceps also can function well as a rotator. This is due to the symmetry of its blades and the leverage gained by the offset shank and handles. The Barton forceps has achieved patronage as an instrumental adjunct for the management of occiput posterior arrests.[1]

The hinged branch is always the anterior one and is applied first. For an oblique posterior position, this can be done either by a direct application over the anterior ear or by the wandering technic. In making a direct application to an ROP, the handle is held in the right hand and the blade is guided by two fingers of the left. The rigid posterior blade is then inserted and applied opposite its mate along the posterior ear, the left hand controlling the handle and the right guiding it into place. The branches are then articulated and the application checked.

The handles are equalized if necessary to correct any asynclytism and the head is flexed. Rotation can be performed with or without the traction bar applied. The handles are turned in the appropriate direction through a wide sweeping arc (Fig. 10-8). This maneuver with the Barton forceps is reminiscent of turning a crank handle. It is usually wise, once rotation has been accomplished, to remove the Barton and apply a classic forceps for the extraction.

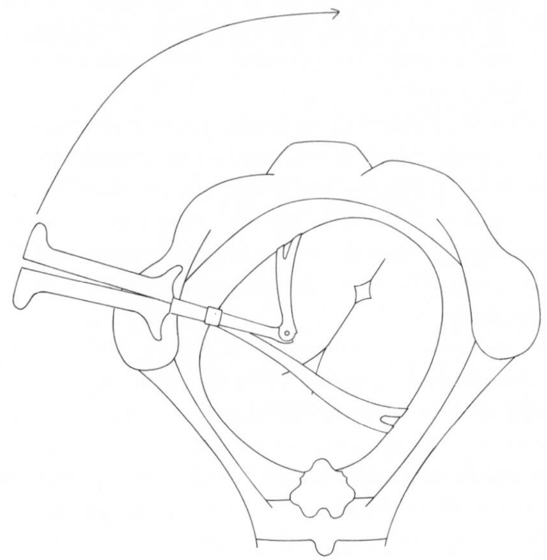

Fig. 10-8. ROP, Barton forceps, application and arc of rotation.

The Barton is uniquely suited for a posterior arrest in a flat pelvis. Rotation in this case should be limited to bringing the sagittal suture to the transverse plane, and extraction is performed in this diameter.

Other Forceps

Other instruments of interest are the forceps of Jacobs,[43] Mann,[62] and Miseo.[65] Their respective instruments have selective hinged blades or shanks and handles so that rotation can be performed, the instrument adjusted, and then the delivery completed. The intent of the designers was to avoid the double application of forceps necessary to perform the modified Scanzoni maneuver. New modifications of traditional instruments, such as Smith's, continue to appear but as yet none have achieved widespread popularity.

Chapter Eleven

Brow and Face Presentations

Together brow and face presentations comprise less than .5 per cent of all deliveries. Most authorities believe that brow presentation is usually a transition between full flexion to a vertex or full extension to a face. The primary etiologic factors which lead to these malpresentations are prematurity, cephalopelvic disproportion, multiparity, and fetal anomalies. The first two conditions may seem paradoxical; however, it is easy to visualize a small infant in a large pelvis not having to undergo total body flexion in order to pass through the pelvic canal. On the other hand, a contracted pelvis or a large baby in a normal pelvis can predispose to brow and face presentation. The pendulus or markedly relaxed abdomen of a multipara can permit the uterus to sag forward, promoting extension of the fetal thoracic and cervical spine. This changes the relationship of the fetal axis to the birth canal and promotes extension of the head. The most common anomaly which presents as a brow or face is anencephaly because of the faulty development of the cranium.

A multiplicity of other possible etiologic factors such as low-lying placenta, tumors of the pelvis, hydramnios, and increased extensor tone of fetal back and neck muscles also have been indicted in various reports.

Current concepts in the management of brow and face presentation stress the liberalization of cesarean section. Conversion maneuvers such as the Thorne, DeLee, and Ziegenspeck have been discarded and version restricted to a second twin or a small deformed baby.[32] Posner et al.[77,78] have demonstrated a high rate of vaginal delivery by following a course of conservative management. Although cesarean section is preferable to a difficult midforceps rotation and extraction of a brow or a face, there remains a significant number of cases which can be managed with forceps.

BROW PRESENTATION

Most brow presentations are transitional and will convert to a face or an occiput. When a brow presentation is diagnosed, the attendant must be certain that no disproportion exists; otherwise, cesarean section is the immediate procedure of choice. Ultraconservatism is the keynote of management, and this is typified by early intervention with cesarean section. The residual few cases which demonstrate progress with labor and are amenable to management with forceps is only about 25 per cent. These usually are the smaller infants in a large pelvis.

The mechanism of labor in those cases which will deliver vaginally is for the brow to assume an anterior position with the occiput filling the hollow of the sacrum. Delivery of the head is accomplished by flexion rather than extension, with the brow, anterior fontanelle, vertex, and occiput sequentially passing over the perineum. The second stage is quite prolonged because of the great expulsive force necessary to accomplish delivery. It is in these instances that forceps and a liberal episiotomy are of great value.

Forceps operations should be approached with great temerity and restricted to those cases in which the brow is not behind the transverse diameter of the pelvis. The Kielland forceps is the instrument of choice. Its long blades with their spacious posterior segment are adaptable to the fronto-occipital diameter of the head. The Kielland's ability to effectively function for rotation and traction reduces the amount of operative manipulation necessary to accomplish delivery.

When applied to an anterior brow presentation, the Kielland is inverted for insertion. The directional markers are oriented toward the posterior fontanelle. The insertion and application are performed in the same manner as for an occiput posterior position. The handles should be slightly elevated rather than depressed for locking the branches in order to allow the blades to obtain a better fit on the parietal bosses. The relationship of the forceps to the head, however, is quite different than with an occiput posterior. The brow with its caput occupies the space between the heels of the blades and the anterior fontanelle is just beneath the shanks (Fig. 11-1). When the Kielland is applied by this technic, the operator must remain aware that the pelvic curve of the blades is inverted.

Once locked, the handles should be elevated to encourage flexion of the head. This maneuver can be repeated to accomplish complete conversion to an occiput posterior, which is recommended by many authorities. On the other hand, conversion to a face can be attempted by repeatedly depressing the handles to encourage extension of the head. According to Moore and Dennen, the majority of brow presentations suitable for vaginal delivery can be converted to occiput posteriors.

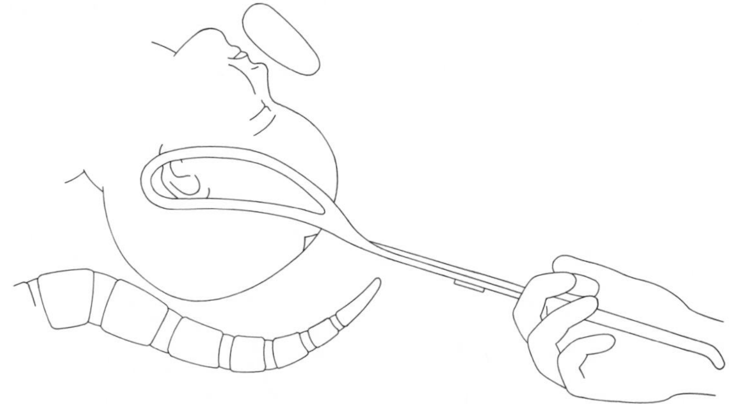

Fig. 11-1. Brow anterior, Kielland forceps application.

Rotation from an oblique diameter such as a left fronto-anterior is performed through a narrow arc as with other Kielland rotations. Traction is downward, to capitalize on the Kielland construction, and a liberal posterolateral episiotomy is indicated to compensate for the overdistention of the perineum produced by the posterior occiput.

FACE PRESENTATION

Face presentations are usually diagnosed earlier than brows due to their distinctive feel on vaginal examination. Since they have a higher incidence of vaginal delivery, they are allowed to labor as long as progress is being made and any degree of pelvic contracture has been excluded. Labor is usually prolonged and frequently internal rotation is delayed until the face reaches and sometimes distends the pelvic floor. As with a brow presentation, the mechanism of delivery is flexion of the fetal head. The presenting chin must be anterior and its undersurface impinge against the symphysis. Delivery is begun with the chin and mouth followed by the nose, eyes, brow, and occiput. Fortunately, only one-third of all face presentations have the chin posterior, and the majority of these spontaneously rotate. Arrested mentum posteriors, however, are best handled by cesarean section. Face presentations in a spacious pelvis frequently surprise the attendant by the ease with which they deliver spontaneously or can be handled with forceps.

The use of forceps should be limited, as with brow presentations, to those cases in which the chin is not behind the transverse diameter of the pelvis. The Kielland forceps is again the instrument of choice, not only for its spacious blades which fit the long diameters of the head so well but for its ability to provide rotation and axis-traction. When rotation is not necessary, however, a classic instrument is perfectly acceptable and preferred by many.

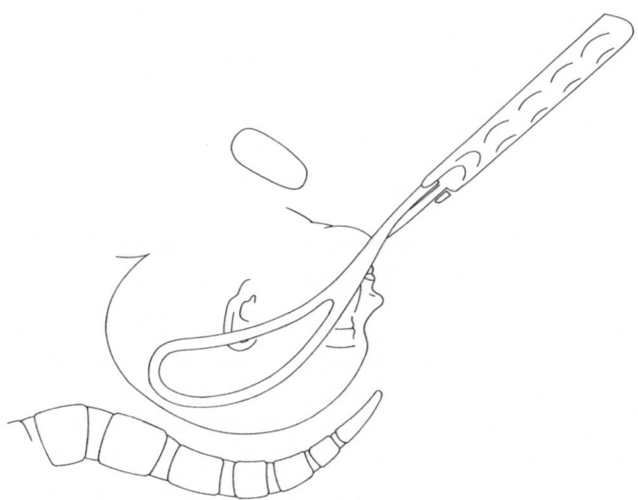

Fig. 11-2. Mentum anterior, Simpson forceps application.

One must remember when using forceps for a face presentation that the focal point of orientation is the chin rather than the occiput. The blades are applied along the mento-occipital diameter of the head. With a classic forceps, the mentum is between the heels of the blades and the face beneath the level of the shanks (Fig. 11-2). With the Kielland forceps, the directional markers .point to the chin rather than the occiput.

For a mentum anterior, the branches of the Kielland are applied as with a classic instrument. Therefore the left blade is applied to the right side of the head and the right to the left side. The handles should be elevated rather then depressed for articulation to achieve a better fit of the blades on the parietal bosses and to prevent slippage. Once locked, the handles are lowered to increase extension of the head. Because of the bayonet shape of the forceps, the heels of the blades are level with the supraorbital ridges and the mouth and nose are above the level of the shanks (Fig. 11-3).

To accomplish delivery of a face presentation with Kielland forceps, downward traction is maintained until the chin is born beneath the symphysis. The handles are then gradually elevated toward the horizontal to accomplish flexion and allow the occiput to deliver over the perineum.

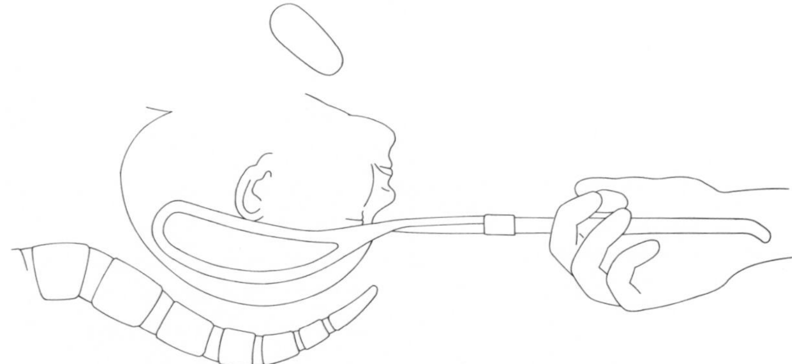

Fig. 11-3. Mentum anterior, Kielland forceps application.

In mentum transverse positions, the chin is still the point of orientation. Therefore an LMT can be handled as an LOT. The classic or inversion method with the Kielland is the preferred technic. The forceps is externally oriented and the right or anterior branch inserted first. It is inverted and inserted beneath the symphysis and cervix into the lower uterine segment. Rotation of the anterior branch is counterclockwise away from the chin. The left or posterior branch is then inserted directly posterior and the shanks are locked. Rotation of an LMT is performed counterclockwise to bring the chin directly anterior. The application is checked, adjusted if necessary, and then the handles are depressed. The latter maneuver assures complete extension of the head prior to instituting traction.

If the operator desires, the Kielland or the Kielland-Barton forceps can be applied to a mentum transverse by the wandering technic. For an RMT, the branches are reversed and rotation is performed in a clockwise direction. This procedure should not be attempted, however, unless the head is near the pelvic floor.

Although many face presentations—and a few brow presentations—can deliver vaginally and be assisted with forceps, cesarean section must still be considered as the primary operative procedure in the management of these cases. The rare instance of a successful manual conversion maneuver or version and extraction should not influence the attendant's basic approach to the problem. Failed conversion maneuvers, complex forceps rotations and extractions, and difficult versions can only lead to the infliction of major fetal and maternal trauma.

Chapter Twelve

Aftercoming Head Forceps

It has been said that breech presentation is the complication which is the ultimate test of obstetric judgement and skill. Breech presentation occurs in 3–4 per cent of all deliveries and carries a fetal risk 3½–4 times that of a normal vertex presentation. This formidable figure has focused attention on the etiology of breeches and their proper obstetric management.[69,70,86,87]

The primary etiologic factor in breech presentation is prematurity. By performing serial x-ray studies, Weisman demonstrated a 24 per cent incidence from the 13th–20th week of gestation, an 8 per cent incidence from the 28th–30th week, and a final incidence of about 4 per cent at the 40th week. Most authorities agree that the fetus does not become crowded by the uterine walls until about the 32nd week, at which time it adapts to the intrauterine contour. Since the bulk of the breech and flexed extremities represents a larger mass than the cephalic pole, it will usually seek the most spacious part of the uterine cavity. Therefore, most breeches will spontaneously change their polarity during the last few weeks of gestation to make use of the more spacious fundus. This thesis gains considerable credence when one reviews the work of Stevenson,[99] who states, "The position of the implanted placenta in the term or near term human uterus as it indents and alters the ovoid shape of the amniotic sac determines the polarity of the sac independently of the fixed polarity of the containing uterus; functionally the fetus accommodates itself to the shape of the sac, the fetal head seeking its smaller pole and thus the placental implantation site has a determining effect upon the presentation of the fetus." The high incidence of breech presentation associated with hydrocephalus is also in accord with this theory.

Even when the increased perinatal mortality associated with breech presentation is corrected for prematurity, the perinatal loss is still close to four times that of a normal vertex presentation. For this reason some authorities have urged more frequent attempts at external cephalic version. According to Holland[41] and Capon,[17] the major cause of fetal death in breech presentations is the marked increase in tentorial tears with subsequent intracranial hemorrhage. Wulff and his associates in their review of 1,300 cases of breech presentation had a corrected mortality of 3.9 per cent. Intracranial trauma and hemorrhage were responsible for 43 per cent of these deaths.

Although the use of cesarean section has been markedly liberalized, and rightfully so, the majority of breeches are still delivered vaginally. For vaginal delivery to be safe, the obstetrician must carefully evaluate whether it can be performed without trauma to mother and child; he must have a plan for the management of the labor and delivery; and he must be liberal with the use of forceps for the aftercoming head. The prognostic index of Zatuchni and Andros[115, 116] regarding vaginal delivery for breeches and the plan of management for labor and delivery advocated by Hansen[38] and Morgan[68] are worthy of review.

Because of the high incidence of intracranial trauma associated with breech delivery, the attendant must pay special attention to the adversely molded aftercoming head. The prophylactic use of aftercoming head forceps should allow for a carefully controlled extraction of the head and eliminate the need for undue torsion and traction of the fetal neck and body as well as excess force on the head through fundal pressure. Forceps are not to be reserved for the difficult cases only.

Since 1924 when the Piper forceps was introduced, it has been the classic instrument for the management of the aftercoming head. Its tapered, shallow blades with spring-like quality allow for a good fit. The perineal curve within the shanks is advantageous in performing flexion of the head, which is the mechanism of delivery. The Piper's extreme length, however, tends to make the instrument unwieldy. For this reason, the author modified it by shortening the shanks and replacing the conventional handle with a pivot lock and finger grips.

Some obstetricians prefer to use a classic forceps such as the Simpson or Elliott for the aftercoming head. Although acceptable, these instruments lack the advantage of a perineal curve and accentuate extension of the fetal body and neck, increasing the risk of injury. The Hawks-Dennen forceps with angulated shanks and the Kielland forceps, because of its compensated pelvic curve, are perfectly acceptable for the aftercoming head. No matter which instrument is used, the concept of liberalization of prophylactic forceps to the aftercoming head is the prime concern.

Forceps can be applied to the aftercoming head only after the shoulders and arms have been delivered and the head, chin posterior, is well in the pelvis. The cardinal principles in applying forceps to the aftercoming head are: (*1*) the forceps is inserted and applied from below upward; (*2*) the application is a pelvic one, rather than purely cephalic; and (*3*) the mechanism of extraction is flexion of the fetal head accomplished by elevating the handles of the forceps.

PIPER FORCEPS

The left branch of the Piper forceps is always inserted and applied first. This will allow proper locking without recrossing the branches. The infant's body is gently carried on a horizontal plane toward the left (mother's right) side. Usually this maneuver, which makes the approach to the left side of the pelvis more available, is performed

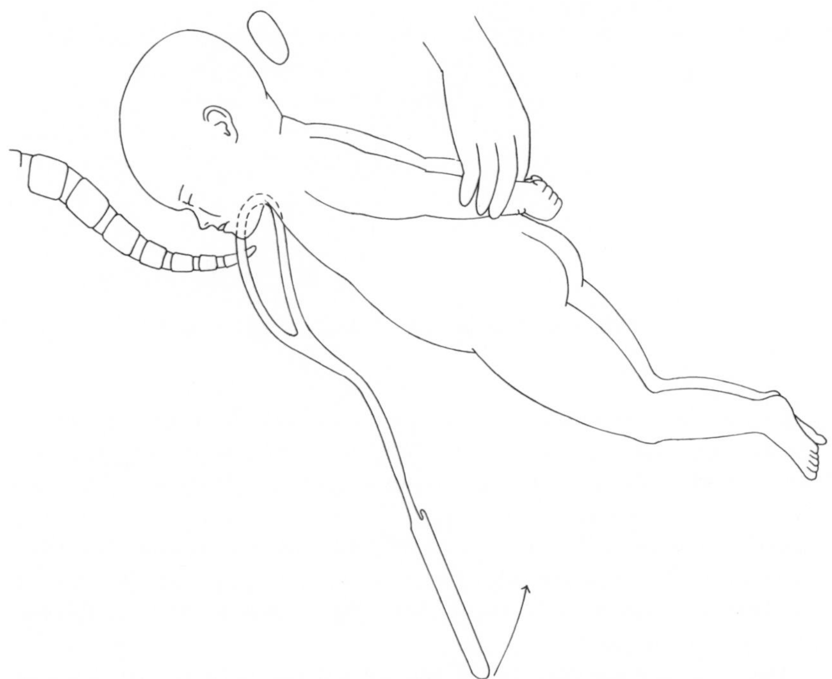

Fig. 12-1. Insertion of left branch, Piper forceps.

by an assistant. The operator should function from beneath the level of the infant's body, which is best accomplished from a kneeling or sitting position.

The left branch is held in the left hand beneath the horizontal and toward the maternal right thigh. The toe of the blade is directed upward toward the left side of the pelvis. Insertion is accomplished by the left hand elevating the handle upward and toward the midline in a sweeping arc while the fingers of the right hand protect the left vaginal wall and guide the blade along the right side of the infant's head (Fig. 12-1). As the handle approaches the midline, the blade will have attained a position in the pelvis alongside the fetal head.

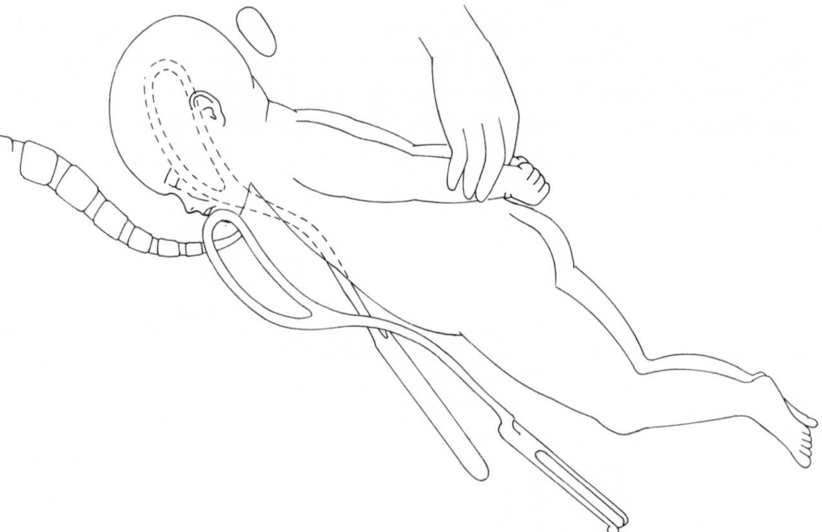

Fig. 12-2. Insertion of right branch, Piper forceps.

The infant's body is now moved by the assistant horizontally toward the mother's left thigh so the right branch can be inserted and applied. This is performed in a similar manner as with the left branch but now the hands are reversed (Fig. 12-2). If there is any resistance to the insertion, the blade should be removed and reinsertion attempted more posteriorly. Appropriate adjustment of insertion and application of the branches also must be made if the head tends toward an oblique diameter of the pelvis.

The branches are now locked and the infant's body returned to the midline and allowed to straddle the shanks of the forceps. The forceps are controlled by the right hand. The handles are grasped from below with the palm turned up and the middle finger in the crotch of the shanks (Fig. 12-3). The right thumb can assist by holding the right thigh of the infant over the shanks. The left hand assists by controlling the fetal body and neck, which is accomplished by the index and middle fingers straddling and splinting the neck.

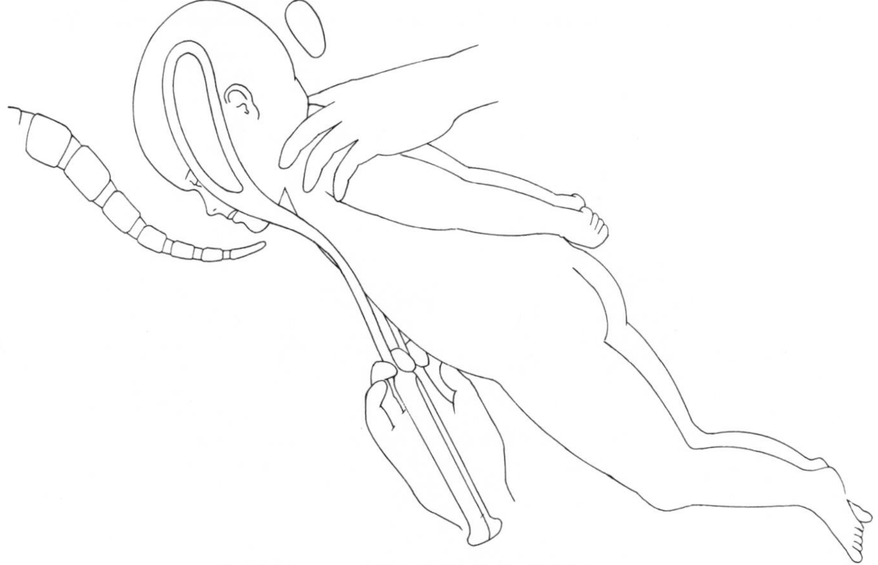

Fig. 12-3. Traction, Piper forceps.

As traction is instituted, the handles of the forceps are gently elevated to encourage flexion of the head. This must be performed slowly if trauma is to be avoided as the suboccipital region passes under the pubic arch. If the operator encounters resistance, he must desist from continuing to elevate the handles. The branches of the forceps should now be gently lowered and traction and elevation of the handles reinstituted. This maneuver can be repeated and will increase flexion of the head, allowing it to deliver over the perineum. Delivery is usually completed with the forceps still applied as the handles pass upward through the horizontal plane. Care must be taken so the head does not drop between the blades as it is extracted.

SHORT PIPER FORCEPS

The variations in technic with the use of the short Piper forceps are a direct reflection of its construction. Since it has a pivot rather than a crossed locking mechanism, either branch may be inserted first. Insertion and application is performed from below, as with the classic Piper. The abbreviated length of the instrument, however, reduces the arc each branch must describe to be applied.

Once both branches have been inserted and applied, the pivot lock is engaged. The forceps is controlled from below by the right hand so that the index and fourth finger hook over the finger grips and the middle finger is between the shanks. Since there are no handles, the infant's abdomen may rest in the palm of the right hand (Fig. 12-4).

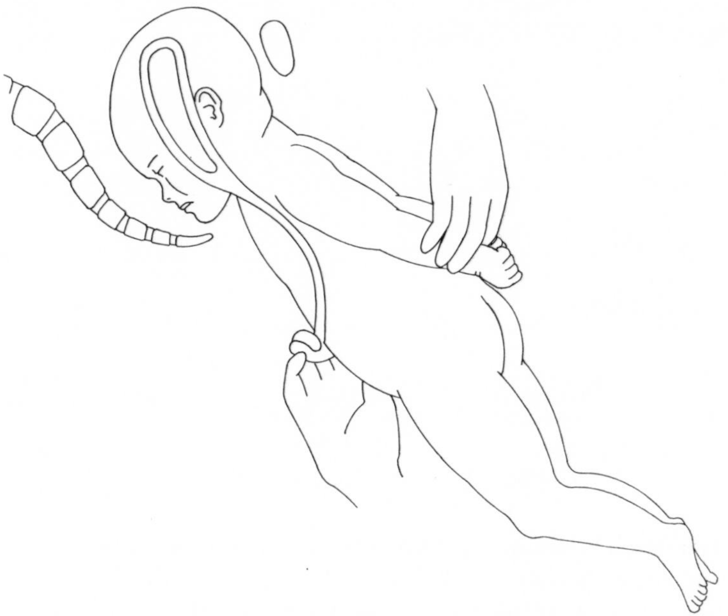

Fig. 12-4. Traction, short Piper forceps.

The left hand functions in aiding control of the fetal body and neck as with the use of the long Piper. Delivery of the head is performed by exerting simultaneous traction and elevation of the finger grips.

Aftercoming head forceps are not to be reserved for the difficult cases or used only when the head is not well in the pelvis. It must be emphasized that the use of prophylactic forceps for the aftercoming head is just as important as the use of prophylactic outlet forceps.

References

1. Anderson, D. G.: Arrested occiput posterior positions. *Clin. Obstet. Gynec. 8*:867, 1965.
2. Aveling, J. H.: *The Chamberlens and the Midwifery Forceps: Memorials of the Family and an Essay on the Invention of the Instrument.* London, Churchill, 1882.
3. Bachman, C.: The Barton obstetrical forceps; a review of its use in fifty-five cases. *Surg. Gynec. Obstet. 45*:805, 1927
4. Barton, L. G., Caldwell, W. E., and Studdiford, W. E., Sr.: A new obstetric forceps. *Amer. J. Obstet. Gynec. 15*:16, 1928.
5. Baxter, J.: Obstetrical forceps; controlled axis traction. *J. Obstet. Gynaec. Brit. Comm. 53*:42, 1946.
6. Bednoff, S. L., and Thomas, B. E.: Brow presentation. *New York J. Med. 67*:803, 1967.
7. Bell, B.: *A System of Surgery,* Vol. XI, 3rd ed. Edinburgh, Charles Elliott, 1789.
8. Bill, A. H.: Forceps rotation of the head in persistent occiput posterior positions. *Amer. J. Obstet. Gynec. 68*:791, 1918.
9. Bill, A. H.: A new axis-traction handle for solid blade forceps. *Amer. J. Obstet. Gynec. 9*:606, 1925.
10. Bill, A. H.: The treatment of the vertex occiput posterior position. *Amer. J. Obstet. Gynec. 26*:615, 1931.
11. Bill, A. H.: Forceps delivery. *Amer. J. Obstet. Gynec. 68*:245, 1954.

11a. Boerma, N. J. A. F.: Eine neve Geburtszange. *Zbl. Gynaek. 11*:565, 1907.

12. Borell, U., and Fernstrom, I.: The mechanism of labour in face and brow, presentation, a radiological study. *Acta Obstet. Gynec. Scand. 39*:626, 1960.
13. Caldeyro-Barcia, R., Alvarez, H., and Reynolds, S. R. M.: A better understanding of uterine contractility through simultaneous recording with an internal and a seven channel external method. *Surg. Gynec. Obstet. 91*:641, 1950.
14. Caldeyro-Barcia, R., and Poserio, J.: Oxytocin and contractility of the pregnant human uterus. *Ann. NY Acad. Sci. 75*:813, 1959.
15. Calkins, L. A.: Occiput posterior-normal presentations. *Amer. J. Obstet. Gynec. 43*:277, 1942.
16. Calkins, L. A.: Occipitoposterior presentation. *Obstet. Gynec. 1*:466, 1953.
17. Capon, N. B.: Intracranial traumata in the newborn. *J. Obstet. Gynaec. Brit. Comm. 29*:572, 1922.

18. Cutter, I. S., and Viets, H. R.: *A Short History of Midwifery.* Philadelphia, Saunders, 1964.
19. Danforth, D. N.: Method of forceps rotation in persistent occiput posterior. *Amer. J. Obstet. Gynec. 65:*120, 1953.
20. Danforth, D. N., and Ellis, A. H.: Midforceps delivery—a vanishing art? *Amer. J. Obstet. Gynec. 86:*29, 1963.
21. Danforth, D. N.: Transverse arrest. *Clin. Obstet. Gynec. 8:*854, 1965.
22. Das, K. N.: *Obstetric Forceps; Its History and Evolution.* St. Louis, Mosby, 1929.
22a. DeLee, J. B.: The prophylactic forceps operation. *Amer. J. Obst. Gynec. 1:*34, 1920.
23. DeLee, J. B.: The treatment of occiput posterior position after engagement of the head. *Surg. Gynec. Obstet. 46:*696, 1928.
24. DeLee, J. B.: and Greenhill, J. P.: *Principles and Practice of Obstetrics,* 9th ed. Philadelphia, Saunders, 1948.
25. Dennen, E. H.: A new forceps with a traction curve. *Amer. J. Obstet. Gynec. 22:*258, 1931.
26. Dennen, E. H.: *Forceps Deliveries,* 2nd ed. Philadelphia, Davis, 1964.
27. Dennen, E. H.: Techniques of application for low forceps. *Clin. Obstet. Gynec. 8:*834, 1965.
28. Dill, L. V.: *The Obstetric Forceps.* Springfield, Ill., Thomas, 1953.
29. Dossert, F. C.: *The Barton Forceps.* New York, Chazy Free Press, 1949.
30. Douglas, R. G., and Stromme, W. B.: *Operative Obstetrics.* New York, Appleton, 1957.
31. Dyer, I.: Trial and failed forceps. *Clin. Obstet. Gynec. 8:*914, 1965.
32. Eastman, N. J., and Hellman, L. M.: *Williams Obstetrics,* 13th ed. New York, Appleton, 1961.
33. Farabeuf, L. H., and Varnier, H.: *Introduction a L'etude clinique et a la Pratique des Accouchements.* Paris, G. Steinheil. 1891.
34. Fleming, A. R., Brandeberry, K. R., and Pearse, W. H.: Introduction of a metric forceps. *Amer. J. Obstet. Gynec. 78:*125, 1959.
35. Foundation for Medical Research: *Perinatal Study.* Philadelphia, 1964.
36. Fuldner, R. V.: Labor complication and cerebral palsy. *Amer. J. Obstet. Gynec. 74:*159, 1957.
37. Hall, J. E., and Kohl, S.: Breech presentation; a study of 1,456 cases. *Amer. J. Obstet. Gynec. 72:*977, 1956.
38. Hansen, E. M.: Breech presentation. *Amer. J. Obstet. Gynec. 41:*575, 1941.
39. Haynes, D. M.: Occiput posterior position. *J.A.M.A. 156:*494, 1954.
40. Hellman, L. M., Epperson, J. W. W., and Connolly, F.: Face and brow presentation. *Amer. J. Obstet. Gynec. 59:*831, 1950.
41. Holland, E.: Cranial stress in the foetus during labour and on the effects of excessive stress on the intracranial contents; with an analysis of 81 cases of torn tentorium cerebilli and subdural cerebral haemorrhage. *J. Obstet. Gynaec. Brit. Comm. 29:*549, 1922.
42. Holland, E., and Bourne, A.: *British Obstetric and Gynaecological Practise.* Philadelphia, Davis, 1955.

43. JACOBS, J. B.: Persistent occipitoposterior; a simple and safe method of treatment with the use of new forceps. *Southern Med. J. 29:*891, 1936.

43a. JACOBSON, A. C.: Evolution in axis-traction. An advance upon the method of utilizing the principle of axis-traction in vogue in obstetric practice unimproved since its introduction by Tarnier in 1877. *Amer. J. Obstet. 35:*326, 1906.

44. KARLSON, S.: On the motility of the uterus during labour and the influence of the motility pattern on the duration of the labour. *Acta Obstet. Gynec. Scand. 28:*209, 1949.

45. KELLY, J. V.: Instrument delivery and the fetal heart rate. *Amer. J. Obstet. Gynec. 87:*529, 1963.

46. KELLY, J. V., and SINES, G.: An assessment of the compression and traction forces of obstetrical forceps. *Amer. J. Obstet. Gynec. 96:*521, 1966.

47. KENWICK, A. N.: Face and brow presentation. *Amer. J. Obstet. Gynec. 66:*67, 1953.

48. KIELLAND, C.: Uber die Anlegung der Zange am nichit notierten Kopf mit beschreibung eines neuen Zangermodelles, und einer neuen Anlegungsmethode. *Monatschr. f. Geburtsh. u. Gynak. 43:*48, 1916.

49. KING, E. L., HERRING, J. S., and KING, J. A.: Modification of the Scanzoni rotation in the management of persistent occipitoposterior positions. *Amer. J. Obstet. Gynec. 61:*872, 1951.

50. KING, E. L.: *Occiput Posterior Positions.* Springfield, Ill., Thomas, 1957.

51. KRISTELLAR: *Monastsschr. Geburtsh. u. Frauenk. 17:*166, 1861.

52. KUTCIPAL, R. A.: Persistent occiput posterior position. *Obstet. Gynec. 14:*296, 1959.

53. LABRECK, F. A.: Obstetric delivery forceps. *Amer. J. Surg. 48:*697, 1940.

54. LAUFE, L. E.: New obstetric forceps. *Obstet. Gynec. 7:*91, 1956.

55. LAUFE, L. E.: The Kielland-Barton (K-B) obstetric forceps. *Obstet. Gynec. 14:*541, 1959.

56. LAUFE, L. E.: An improved Piper forceps. *Obstet. Gynec. 29:*284, 1967.

57. LAUFE, L. E.: A new divergent outlet forceps. *Amer. J. Obstet. Gynec. 101:*509, 1968.

58. LUIKART, R.: A modification of the Kielland, Simpson and Tucker-McLane forceps to simplify their use and improve function and safety. *Amer. J. Obstet. Gynec. 34:*686, 1937.

59. LUIKART, R.: A new forceps possessing a sliding lock, modified fenestra, with improved handle and axis-traction attachment. *Amer. J. Obstet. Gynec. 40:*1058, 1940.

60. MACARTHUR, J. S.: Reduction of the hazards of breech presentation by external cephalic version. *Amer. J. Obstet. Gynec. 88:*302, 1964.

61. MCINTIRE, M. S., and PEARSE, W. H.: Follow-up evaluation of infants delivered by electronically recorded forceps delivery. *Amer. J. Obstet. Gynec. 89:*540. 1964.

62. MANN, J.: The application of a universal joint to obstetric forceps. *Amer. J. Obstet. Gynec. 26:*399, 1933.

63. *Manual of Standards in Obstetric—Gynecologic Practice.* 2nd ed. Chicago, A.C.O.G., 1965.
64. Maughan, G. B.: Safe and simple delivery of persistent posterior and transverse positions. *Amer. J. Obstet. Gynec. 71:*741, 1956.
65. Miseo, A.: New obstetric forceps with a split universal joint principle. *Obstet. Gynec. 8:*487, 1956.
66. Mishell, D., and Kelly, J. V.: The obstetrical forceps and the vacuum extractor: an assessment of their compressive force. *Obstet. Gynec. 19:* 204, 1962.
67. Moore, E. J. T., and Dennen, E. H.: Management of persistent brow presentations. *Obstet. Gynec. 6:*186, 1955.
68. Morgan, H. S.: The management of breech presentation. *Clin. Obstet. Gynec. 5:*1009, 1962.
69. Morgan, H. S., and Kane, S. H.: Analysis of 16,327 breech births. *J.A.M.A. 187:*262, 1964.
70. Morley, G. W.: Breech presentation—a 15-year review. *Obstet. Gynec. 30:*745, 1967.
71. Murchan, R. R.: New obstetric maneuver for dystocia. *J.A.M.A. 155:* 1442, 1955.
72. Patterson, S. P., Mulliniks, R. C., Jr., and Schreier, P. C.: Breech presentation in the primigravida. *Amer. J. Obstet. Gynec. 98:*1967.
73. Pearse, W. H.: Electronic recording of forceps delivery. *Amer. J. Obstet. Gynec. 86:*43, 1963.
74. Pearse, W. H.: Forceps versus spontaneous delivery. *Clin. Obstet. Gynec. 8:*813, 1965.
75. Pearse, W. H.: Personal communication, April, 1967.
76. Piper, E. B., and Bachman, C.: The prevention of fetal injuries in breech delivery. *J.A.M.A. 92:*217, 1929.
77. Posner, A. C., Friedman, S., and Posner, L. B.: Modern trends in the management of face and brow presentations. *Surg. Gynec. Obstet. 104:* 485, 1957.
78. Posner, L. B., Rubin, E. J., and Posner, A. C.: Face and brow presentation; a continuing study. *Obstet. Gynec. 21:*745, 1963.
79. Puddicombe, J. F.: Maternal posture for correction of posterior fetal position. *J. Int. Coll. Surg. 23:*73, 1955.
80. Reddoch, J. W.: Management of occipito-posterior positions with special reference to Scanzoni maneuver. *South. Med. J. 27:*615, 1934.
81. Reddoch, J. W.: Face presentation. *Amer. J. Obstet. Gynec. 56:*86, 1948.
82. Reynolds, S. R. M., Head, O. O., Bruns, P., and Hellman, L. M.: A multi-channel strain-gage tokodynamometer: an instrument for studying patterns of uterine contractions in pregnant women. *Bull. Hopkins Hosp. 82:*446, 1948.
83. Reynolds, S. R. M.: *Physiology of the Uterus with Clinical Correlations,* 2nd ed. New York. Hoeber, 1949.
84. Reynolds, S. R. M., Harris, J. S., and Kaiser, I. H.: *Clinical Measurement of Uterine Forces in Pregnancy and Labor.* Springfield, Ill., Thomas, 1954.

85. RIEDIGER, L.: Ein Schloss fur die Kiellandzange zur Entwicklung toter Kinder nach vorausgegangen Perforation. *Zentralbl. fur Gynak. 51:* 2198, 1927.
86. RUBIN, A., and GRIMM, G.: Results in breech presentation: a 7-year study. *Amer. J. Obstet. Gynec. 86:*1048, 1963.
87. RUBIN, A.: Birth injuries: incidence, mechanisms, and end results. *Obstet. Gynec. 23:*218, 1964.
88. RUSSELL, K. P., and FRANKEL, I. V.: Forceps in common usage. *Clin. Obstet. Gynec. 8:*822, 1965.
89. SAVAGE, J. E.: Forceps delivery. *Clin. Obstet. Gynec. 4:*917, 1958.
90. SCANZONI, F. W.: *Lehrbuch der Geburtshulfe,* 2nd ed. Vienna, Seidel, 1853.
91. SEIDES, S.: A "two-forceps maneuver" for persistent occipitoposterior presentation. *Surg. Gynec. Obstet. 36:*421, 1923.
92. SHUTE, W. B.: An obstetrical forceps which uses a new principle of parallelism. *Amer. J. Obstet. Gynec. 77:*442, 1959.
93. SKALLY, T. W., and KRAMER, T. F.: Brow presentation. *Obstet. Gynec. 15:*616, 1960.
94. SMELLIE, W.: *Treatise on the Theory and Practice of Midwifery.* London, The New Sydenham Society, 1876.
95. SMITH, E. C.: A new obstetric forceps for rotation and extraction of the fetal head in a single application. *Amer. J. Obstet. Gynec. 94:*931, 1966.
96. *Soranus' Gynecology,* translated with an introduction by O. Temkin, with the assistance of N. J. Eastman, L. Edelstein, and A. F. Guttmacher. Baltimore, The Johns Hopkins Press, 1956.
97. SPEERT, H.: Obstetric forceps. *Clin. Obstet. Gynec. 3:*761, 1960.
98. STEER, C. M.: *Moloy's Evaluation of the Pelvis in Obstetrics,* 2nd ed Philadelphia, Saunders, 1959.
99. STEVENSON, C. S.: Principle cause of breech presentation in single term pregnancies. *Amer J. Obstet. Gynec. 60:*641, 1950.
100. STUDDIFORD, W. E.: *The Barton Forceps.* New York, Sklar Manufacturing Company, 1946.
101. TARNIER: Le nouveau forceps de M. Tarnier. *Progr. Med. 5:*146, 1877.
102. TARNIER: Examen du forceps a aiguilles. *Ann. de gynec. 7:*161, 1877.
103. TARNIER: Le forceps de M. Tarnier. *Progr. Med. 6:*517, 1878.
104. THIERRY, E.: Les Spatules Manoeuvre du toboggan (le T.). *La Presse Medicale 68:*317, 1960.
105. ULLERY, J. C., TETERIS, N. J., BOTSCHNER, A. W., and MCDANIELS, B.: Traction and compression forces exerted by obstetric forceps and their effect on fetal heart rate. *Amer. J. Obstet. Gynec. 85:*1066, 1963.
106. WEISMAN, A. I.: Antepartum study of fetal polarity and rotation. *Amer. J. Obstet. Gynec. 48:*550, 1944.
107. WHITACRE, F. E.: Forceps management of breech and face presentations. *Clin. Obstet. Gynec. 8:*882, 1965.
108. WHITE, H. E.: *Physics, An Exact Science.* Princeton, N.J., Van Nostrand, 1959.

109. Willson, J. R.: *Atlas of Obstetric Technic.* St. Louis, Mosby, 1961.

110. Willson, J. R.: *Management of Obstetric Difficulties.* St. Louis, Mosby, 1961.

111. Wright, R. C.: Reduction of perinatal mortality and morbidity in breech delivery through use of Cesarean section. *Obstet. Gynec. 14:*758, 1959.

112. Wulff, G. J., Trueblood, A. C., and Holland, R. A.: Management of the aftercoming head in breech presentation. *Obstet. Gynec. 16:*288, 1960.

113. Wylie, B.: Traction in forceps deliveries. *Amer. J. Obstet. Gynec. 24:* 425, 1935.

114. Wylie, B.: Forceps traction, an index of birth difficulty. *Amer. J. Obstet. Gynec. 86:*38, 1963.

115. Zatuchni, G. I., and Andros, G. J.: Prognostic index for vaginal delivery in breech presentation at term. *Amer. J. Obstet, Gynec. 93:*237, 1965.

116. Zatuchni, G. I., and Andros, G. J.: Prognostic index for vaginal delivery in breech presentation at term. *Amer. J. Obstet. Gynec. 98:*854, 1967.

Index

71 7 6 5 4 3